PSYCHIATRIC ENCOUNTERS

MEDICAL ANTHROPOLOGY: HEALTH, INEQUALITY, AND SOCIAL JUSTICE

Series editor: Lenore Manderson

Books in the Medical Anthropology series are concerned with social patterns of and social responses to ill health, disease, and suffering, and how social exclusion and social justice shape health and healing outcomes. The series is designed to reflect the diversity of contemporary medical anthropological research and writing, and will offer scholars a forum to publish work that showcases the theoretical sophistication, methodological soundness, and ethnographic richness of the field.

Books in the series may include studies on the organization and movement of peoples, technologies, and treatments, how inequalities pattern access to these, and how individuals, communities, and states respond to various assaults on well-being, including those from illness, disaster, and violence.

Jessica Hardin, *Faith and the Pursuit of Health: Cardiometabolic Disorders in Samoa*

Carina Heckert, *Fault Lines of Care: Gender, HIV, and Global Health in Bolivia*

Alison Heller, *Fistula Politics: Birthing Injuries and the Quest for Continence in Niger*

Joel Christian Reed, *Landscapes of Activism: Civil Society, HIV and AIDS Care in Northern Mozambique*

Beatriz M. Reyes-Foster, *Psychiatric Encounters: Madness and Modernity in Yucatan, Mexico*

Sonja van Wichelen, *Legitimating Life: Adoption in the Age of Globalization and Biotechnology*

PSYCHIATRIC ENCOUNTERS

Madness and Modernity in Yucatan, Mexico

BEATRIZ M. REYES-FOSTER

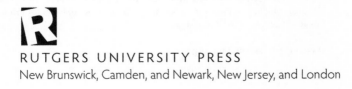

RUTGERS UNIVERSITY PRESS

New Brunswick, Camden, and Newark, New Jersey, and London

Library of Congress Cataloging-in-Publication Data

Names: Reyes-Foster, Beatriz M., author.
Title: Psychiatric encounters : madness and modernity in Yucatan, Mexico /
    Beatriz M. Reyes-Foster.
Description: New Brunswick, New Jersey : Rutgers University Press, [2018] |
    Series: Medical anthropology: health, inequality, and social justice |
    Includes bibliographical references and index.
Identifiers: LCCN 2018005952 | ISBN 9780813594866 (cloth) | ISBN 9780813594859
    (pbk.) | ISBN 9780813594873 (epub) | ISBN 9780813594897 (web PDF)
Subjects: LCSH: Mental health—Social aspects—Mexico. | Mental health
    services—Mexico. | Mayas—Mental health. | Mayas—Psychology.
Classification: LCC RA790.7.M6 R49 2018 | DDC 362.19689—dc23
LC record available at https://lccn.loc.gov/2018005952

A British Cataloging-in-Publication record for this book is available from the
British Library.

www.rutgersuniversitypress.org

Manufactured in the United States of America

For Ron, who lived it; Aydin, who lightened it; Rowan, who kept it going; and Miles, who almost missed it.

And for my mother, Beatriz Cortes Camarillo, who sacrificed many of her own dreams so that I might achieve all of mine.

CONTENTS

Foreword by Lenore Manderson   ix
Note on Text   xiii

1   Introduction: Las Lomas at the Threshold of Modernity   1

2   Coloniality, *La Zona del Estar*, and Yucatan's Maya Heritage   29

3   Making the Matrix   57

4   Modernity: Problem and Promise of Mexican Psychiatry   83

5   Negotiating Truth in the Psychiatric Encounter   110

6   In the Heart of Madness   140

7   Epilogue   165

Acknowledgments   171
Notes   175
Bibliography   181
Index   191

FOREWORD

LENORE MANDERSON

Medical Anthropology: Health, Inequality, Social Justice, a new series from Rutgers University Press, is designed to capture the diversity of contemporary medical anthropological research and writing. The beauty of ethnography is its capacity, through storytelling, to make sense of suffering as a social experience, and to set it in context. Central to our focus in this series on health, illness, and social justice, therefore, is the way in which social structures and ideologies shape the likelihood and impact of infections, injuries, bodily ruptures and disease, chronic conditions and disability, treatment and care, and social repair and death.

The brief for this series is broad. The books are concerned with health and illness, healing practices and access to care, but the authors illustrate, too, the importance of context—of geography, physical condition, service availability, and income. Health and illness are social facts; the circumstances of the maintenance and loss of health are always and everywhere shaped by structural, global, and local relations. Society, culture, economy, and political organization as much as ecology shape the variance of illness, disability, and disadvantage. But as medical anthropologists have long illustrated, the relationships of social context and health status are complex. In addressing these questions, the authors in this series showcase the theoretical sophistication, methodological rigor, and empirical richness of the field, while expanding a map of illness, social, and institutional life to illustrate the effects of material conditions and social meanings in troubling and surprising ways.

The books in the series move across social circumstances, health conditions, and geography—and describe the intersections and interactions of those forces—to demonstrate how individuals, communities, and states manage assaults on well-being. The books reflect medical anthropology as a constantly changing field of scholarship, drawing on diverse research in residential and virtual communities, clinics and laboratories, emergency care and public health settings, with service providers, individual healers and households, and with social bodies, human bodies, and biologies. Although medical anthropology once concentrated on systems of healing, particular diseases, and embodied experiences, today the field has expanded to include environmental disaster and war, science, technology and faith, gender-based violence, and forced migration. Curiosity about the body and its vicissitudes remains a pivot for our work, but our concerns are with the location of bodies in social life, and how social structures, temporal imperatives, and shifting exigencies shape life courses. This dynamic field reflects an ethics of the discipline to address these pressing issues of our time.

Globalization has contributed to and adds to the complexity of influences on health outcomes; it (re)produces social and economic relations that institutionalize poverty, unequal conditions of everyday life and work, and environments in which diseases increase or subside. Globalization patterns the movement and relations of peoples, technologies and knowledge, programs and treatments; it shapes differences in health experience and outcomes across space; it informs and amplifies inequalities at individual and country levels. Global forces and local inequalities compound and constantly load on individuals to impact their physical and mental health, and their households and communities. At the same time, as the subtitle of this series indicates, we are concerned with questions of social exclusion and inclusion, social justice and repair, again both globally and in local settings. The books will challenge readers not only to reflect on sickness and suffering, and deficit and despair, but also on resistance and restitution—how people respond to injustices and evade the fault lines that might seem to predetermine life outcomes. While not all of the books take this direction, the aim is to widen the frame within which we conceptualize embodiment and suffering.

Las Lomas was Yucatan's psychiatric hospital, established in 1978 and charged with leading the process of deinstitutionalization in the state. When Beatriz Reyes-Foster began her anthropological research there, it was dirty and run down; its residents sometimes isolated and restrained, bored and confused. Those with recalcitrant madness, for whom psychotherapy and pharmaceutical treatment had little impact, instead received electroconvulsive therapy. The staff was sometimes indifferent, sometimes belligerent. As the book begins, Las Lomas is described as a "medieval dungeon" of no possibility of appeal or reprieve. Yet with gentle restraint, *Psychiatric Encounters: Madness and Modernity in Yucatan, Mexico*, takes us into this building to engage with its clinicians and the patients: the former committed to the goal of deinstitutionalization and the best possible care—always contestable in the face of health service inefficiencies and staff shortages.

But the problems that beset Las Lomas and its clinicians and patients are far more than this. Originally built beside a rubbish dump on the outskirts of Merida, Yucatan, in one of the poorest states of Mexico, the hospital came to provide care for the poorest and more marginalized of people—not all mad, but confused, hurt, impoverished, and indigent. Most are Maya, and as Reyes-Foster illustrates, indigeneity carves out gross inequalities that complicate everyday life outcomes and the care that might be needed when things go wrong. At the heart of this extraordinary book, Reyes-Foster illustrates how the treatment and experience of madness in Mexico are an outcome of the coloniality of the postrevolutionary state. Both madness and being Maya are antipathetic to state ideas of modernity. To explain this, she draws on a wealth of work of indigenous anthropologists and other social theorists from Mexico and elsewhere: this is genuine writing from the South. Engaging with these refreshing ideas, Reyes-Foster illustrates how social structure and social relations are shaped by concerns about indigeneity and modernity, and how these are refracted through a struggling health care system, perverse health insurance systems, and family discord. As she illustrates, the patients are an end point, but they are also part of Mexico's large and complex neo-colonial bureaucracy and Yucatan's marginal position to it.

NOTE ON TEXT

This ethnographic material was culled from hundreds of hours of participant observation, interviews, field notes, and recordings gathered over eighteen months of research between 2008 and 2013 in Yucatán, Mexico. In the interest of anonymity, the name and exact location of Las Lomas, the psychiatric facility where this research is set, have been disguised. Some quotations from transcripts and field notes have been edited for flow and coherence, but the content has been preserved. The identities of patients and doctors who were able to provide and willingly gave their informed consent to participate in this research have been disguised with pseudonyms to preserve their privacy. Some characters in this book, such as Lina, Silvia, and Doña Isabel, are composite examples based on real people. This is especially the case for patients whom I describe as experiencing psychosis and whose interactions I observed in the context of psychiatric assessment. Although research in the acute ward was approved and granted exempt status by the University of Central Florida Internal Review Board for the Protection of Human Subjects, I took this extra step to further respect the boundaries and dignity of the people whose suffering I witnessed and who likely never knew I was there. All the events I describe in this book happened in the manner described, based on my own field notes or recordings. Most quotations are based on taped conversations, though others are based on field notes taken during or shortly after the encounter described.

PSYCHIATRIC ENCOUNTERS

1 · INTRODUCTION
Las Lomas at the Threshold of Modernity

[Las Lomas] is a medieval dungeon. . . . I would sooner lock my relative in a room than I would allow them to spend one second in your "hospital."
—"J. R.," October 19, 2012

The truth is that colonization, in its very essence, already appeared to be a great purveyor of psychiatric hospitals.
—Frantz Fanon, *The Wretched of the Earth*

In the fall of 2012, after I returned from fieldwork in Mexico, I wrote the first version of what would eventually become the foundation of this book. It was a paper I would present at the 2012 meeting of the American Anthropological Association in San Francisco. On a whim, as I was finishing the paper, I googled the name "Las Lomas." As the search results appeared, a headline grabbed my attention: *Envejece Las Lomas*, "Las Lomas Ages." The brief story—233 words in total—was published on the website of a local paper with a daily print run of about 70,000 copies sold throughout the Yucatan Peninsula. It described the state psychiatric hospital's crumbling infrastructure, noting that the hospital director had publicly announced the need for a new facility. "The life cycle of this hospital has come to an end," the note read. "There is an urgent need for a new construction with a different model and modern technology."

I scrolled down to the comments section and discovered only one, dated October 19 of the same year. Written anonymously by someone who went by the screen name "J. R.," the comment was prefaced with a statement: "copied from an email sent to Juan Vasquez, former director of Las Lomas." The comment continued: "Las Lomas is a prison, a medieval dungeon where people are locked away without the possibility of appeal, denied their liberty following an initial assessment made without seriousness by a recent graduate or student. . . . I would sooner lock a relative of mine in a room in my house before I would ever bring him to your 'hospital.' . . . You do not have the moral authority to lock people up nor tell them what to do or not do with their lives. You have failed." I thought about

J. R.'s comments as I reflected on my most recent experience at Las Lomas—a three-month visit in 2012 during which I had plunged into the guts of this institution more deeply than in the six months of continuous fieldwork I had conducted in 2008 or research I would undertake later. Even as I was finishing a seven-page oral presentation, I had become convinced I would never turn my experiences into a book—writing about my work there had become too emotionally draining. My months inside Las Lomas left a lasting impression, one I carry with me to this day; a sensation of nausea is triggered when I think of the smell of the ward, or hear, in my mind, the sound of desperate cries through open windows. This was *One Flew Over the Cuckoo's Nest* brought to horrible life.

The Las Lomas state psychiatric hospital is similar to many other Mexican public psychiatric hospitals. The international human rights organization Disability Rights International (DRI) has published several reports over the years outlining the horrific conditions of public psychiatric institutions in Mexico (MDRI 2000; DRI 2011, 2015), where people are routinely abandoned to unhygienic conditions, stripped of privacy and dignity, forced to wear uniforms, subjected to physical restraints, and deprived of food, water, and medical care. The most recent report, published in 2015, notes that despite previous reports and public acknowledgment by the Mexican state of the conditions of its psychiatric institutions, DRI investigations have continued to uncover "a pattern of egregious and widespread human rights violations" (2015, i). What I had encountered in my time conducting ethnographic fieldwork resonated with several of the findings in the DRI reports. During my time in the wards at Las Lomas, I witnessed patients restrained for extended periods of time, medicated against their will, and placed in isolation in a room with nothing but an ancient metal hospital bed, a black rubber mattress, and a broken toilet. Patients are forced to wear a uniform, allowed no personal property (not even reading material), and they are without access to a telephone or other means of communication. Conditions inside the wards were horrific: the buildings were literally crumbling around them, with paint peeling off the walls, which were scratched with graffiti and messages from patients who had passed through these rooms. The odors from the constantly broken toilets permeated the entire ward with the stench of human waste. Inside the acute wards, patients were locked in to their dormitories for up to twenty hours a day and allowed out only to consult with the attending psychiatrist, visit with their relatives in the ward vestibule, and eat (also in the ward vestibule). They were never allowed outdoors. When patients are committed—even if they enter the institution on a voluntary basis—they become wards of the state. They cannot leave voluntarily and are essentially at the mercy of the attending psychiatrist. Medieval dungeon, indeed.

Yet I also realized the dungeon masters were not evil people. They were, for the most part, hard-working professionals—psychiatrists, nurses, and social workers—even if they occasionally did not get along with one another. I was reminded of a phrase I saw in an unrelated book on birth in post–Soviet Russia (Rivkin-Fish 2005), a prelude borrowing the words of musician Boris Grebenshikov: "Everything I do is an attempt to live like a human being, in conditions that are inhumane." The people I worked with at Las Lomas—patients and hospital employees alike—seemed to be striving to do just that, to live like human beings under inhumane conditions that seemed to stubbornly persist despite clear recognition by everyone on the ground that the current system simply was not working.

This book is an ethnography of a psychiatric facility in Yucatan, Mexico. Las Lomas, of course, is not its real name. It is a pseudonym chosen to protect, as best I can, the identities of the medical providers and patients who generously allowed me to bear witness to life in a place some would go on to describe as a hell on earth. Las Lomas is a public psychiatric hospital in the southeastern state of Yucatan in Mexico. The stories I will share may be difficult to read—some were extraordinarily difficult to write—but they represent a slice in time, a fraction of ethnographic material collected over several seasons of institutional fieldwork inside the hospital's wards and more than a decade of ethnographic engagement in the region.

The purpose of this research was not to capture the visceral exposure of human suffering, nor to document a pornography of violence, but rather, initially, to understand how users of Mexico's public mental health care services navigated these services. In 2008, my research was focused on the hospital's suicide prevention program, which was part of my broader ethnographic work on suicide. However, as I spent more and more time at Las Lomas, other questions emerged. When I returned to the hospital in 2012, my interests focused on the medical interactions between patients and psychiatrists, residents, and other medical providers.

Nearly ten years after the inception of *Seguro Popular*, the national health care scheme that has come to insure millions of previously uninsured Mexicans, Las Lomas forms part of a vast nationwide network of medical institutions utilized by nearly 55 million people (INEGI 2016). Yet at the same time that Seguro Popular and medical reform promised access to quality medical care for all Mexicans, economists and politicians have fretted over the viability of its health institutions, particularly the *Instituto Mexicano del Seguro Social* (IMSS), colloquially referred to as *el Seguro*, the National Institute for Social Security, which provides health care and retirement benefits to 62 million privately employed citizens (Instituto Nacional De Estadística 2016). IMSS is beloved by some (Hayden 2007) but despised by others—*Seguro? Seguro que te mueres!*[1] (Surety? Surely you will die!) is a popular expression for my interlocutors when talking about el Seguro. The financial viability of IMSS had long been a source of concern in a neoliberal Mexico. In the thirteen years that I have been an active field researcher in Mexico, the neoliberal groundwork laid during President Carlos Salinas de Gortari's *sexenio* in the 1980s has led to the steady privatization of various state enterprises and a definitive move toward free market economics, to the great benefit of some and the harm of others. Some argue that neoliberal economic reforms in the last thirty years have resulted in the emergence of a Mexican middle class and quite likely contributed to the dramatic decrease of migration to the United States (Duncan 2017). At the same time that neoliberal economic reforms have firmly taken root, Mexican state policy and public discourse continues to be dominated, as it has since the nineteenth century, by a concern of *modernity*. How do we make Mexico modern?

Yucatan ranks sixteenth out of thirty-two federative entities (thirty-one states and the Federal District of Mexico City) in poverty in Mexico, with just over 80 percent of the population categorized as living in some kind of economic distress.[2] Some 45.9 percent of the population is said to be living in poverty, with 10.7 percent considered to be in extreme poverty, 27.7 percent considered "vulnerable" to falling into poverty for lack of "social" resources, such as access to quality education, health care, or social security, and 7.0 percent vulnerable to falling into poverty because of low income (CONEVAL 2014). While Latin American intellectuals like Nestor García Canclini (1989) and his predecessors such as Octavio Paz ([1950] 1993) and José Vasconcelos ([1979] 1997) wrote of Mexican modernities, cosmic races, and hybrid cultures, the values they attached to modernity—progressive, technological, efficient—betray a vision of modernity congruent with the Global North.[3] Although the way modernity itself has been defined has changed over time, concerns voiced in public opinion columns in 2016 echo those of the past. Despite reform, Mexico continues to be plagued by political corruption, economic disparities, and financial stagnation, all seen as emblematic obstacles to realizing this vision.

One Flew Over the Cuckoo's Nest (Forman 1975) occupies a special place in the U.S. imagination as an epitome of the horrors of psychiatric institutionalization. Having grown up in the United States, this film became a point of reference as I began to process what I witnessed in the wards in Yucatan. In my interactions with people unaffiliated with the hospital, my disclosure of my project and my work inside the institution was invariably met with a grimace: "You're working *where*?" Occasionally this was followed by gallows humor admonishing me to be careful, lest they decide to keep me. While *One Flew Over the Cuckoo's Nest* does not have the same salience in Mexico, local imaginaries of the *manicomio* (asylum) and its inhabitants exist. These imaginaries can be summed up in a single word: *locura* (madness).

MADNESS

Eva was a recent chemistry graduate from the local state university. She had gotten a job as a laboratory technician at one of the university's research laboratories. Her family—her mother and unwed siblings—lived in Chelem, a nearby beach community. Eva's new job meant she could now live on her own and no longer had to make the forty-minute commute back to her hometown every day. It also meant her family now saw her as someone who could contribute financially to the household, even though her earnings were meager. Eva shared this view— she had made a promise to her father shortly before his death that she would complete her studies and become a professional in order to help pull her family out of poverty. However, things did not go as planned: shortly after Eva started working, her mother, now a widow, and one of her sons-in-law became embroiled in an ugly legal dispute that split the family into two sides. Soon, both sides were pressuring her to support one or the other. Her brother-in-law asked Eva to testify in court against her mother, something that greatly distressed her.

Soon, Eva began to research things obsessively on the Internet, as she was convinced that numbers and dates held hidden meanings. Although she considered herself a skeptical scientist, she began to think her sister had cursed her hand, causing her spasmic pain. The day she was scheduled to testify, her brother-in-law sent her a text message saying he was sending someone to pick her up. Eva panicked, suddenly fearful that the person who was coming was going to hurt her. She left her apartment and asked a friend to help her hide. Soon, her friend realized that something was very wrong. Eva was hearing voices and speaking incoherently. Her friend contacted Eva's mother, who saw her daughter's mental state and took her to Las Lomas, where she was involuntarily committed.

A few days after she was hospitalized, Eva sat in a consultation room inside the acute ward. Her attending psychiatrist, Dr. Maria Tun, had been closely monitoring her progress, and was pleased to see that many of Eva's symptoms had remitted.

"Can you tell us what happened?" Dr. Tun asked Eva, a question she asked her each day.

Eva put her fingers over the bridge of her nose and squeezed her eyes shut. "*Todo parecía locura* [it was all like madness]," she began, "people I knew suddenly frightened me. Things I saw on the internet suddenly seemed connected to one another, like, dates and times and astrological events. I thought I was being watched. I thought my hand was cursed and my food was being poisoned."

Eva's vivid description is a small window into the experience of psychosis. The way she begins her story is meaningful: *todo parecía locura* (it all seemed like madness). Madness, for Eva, signified a frightening state of blurred boundaries between reality and fantasy, what Janis Jenkins (2015) calls "the edge of experience."

Madness, writes Tanya Luhrmann, is terrifying (Luhrmann 2016). It blurs the defining features of personhood, reminding us "that the foundations of our being are built on sand" (270). The suffering of people who are seen as mad is a stark reminder of the fragility of the human psyche. Las Lomas frightens because of the people it houses, people broadly conceived in Mexican society as *los locos* (the mad). Madness troubles us, and it troubles most Mexicans, because it so easily distorts what we believe makes us human. For Eva, the fragility of her own sanity—her rapid transformation from an educated young scientist to a frightened, delusional human being—illustrates how madness is simultaneously alien to our everyday experience yet closer than any of us care to admit.

Mental illness, particularly what some call madness (those forms of severe mental illness that necessitate confinement in a psychiatric institution) is as stigmatized in Mexico as it is in the United States—although, as I will discuss, the etiology of severe mental illness and other kinds of mental distress is understood and addressed differently on the local level. In this book, I frequently use the word "madness" to describe the symptoms and experiences of the people I interacted with. I do this because madness is a more open-ended term than "mental illness," "schizophrenia," or "psychosis." It is a kind of catchall term that describes a swath of symptoms, from delusions to hallucinations to crippling melancholy. It provides us with continuity: when I write of madness I write of it the same way as do some of my intellectual interlocutors—Fanon ([1952] 2008, [1961] 2004), Luhrmann (2016), Ríos Molina (2009). The word "madness" (locura in Spanish) resists the sanitizing effects of medicalization and burrows in its contrarian roots, showing the messiness of human suffering that accompanies it. As I discuss later in this chapter, what makes a person "mad" or "loco" in this context is not a medical diagnosis but socially determined; the term is both troubling and flexible.

While Yucatan has frequently been portrayed by regional specialists as a "world apart [from the rest of Mexico]" (Moseley and Terry 1980; Terry et al. 2010), a culturally distinct area with ties closer to the Caribbean and Europe than to central Mexico, it remains firmly part of the Mexican state, intertwined within the nation's own historical narrative. The history of psychiatry in Yucatan and Mexico is characterized by cycles where a new method supplants an old one in the name of modernity (Sacristán 2005). Before Las Lomas, people with mental illness were housed at the old Hospital Leandro León Ayala, usually referred to as the Asilo Ayala, a beautiful building that today houses Bellas Artes, the state school of fine arts. Inaugurated on February 6, 1906, the old Asilo Ayala and the former penitentiary and still-operating Hospital O'Horan were commissioned by President Porfirio Diaz, whose thirty-five-year dictatorship is today remembered as El Porfiriato (the Porfirate or Porfirian period, roughly from 1876–1911). Porfirian development policy was inspired by a Comptian-influenced positivist philosophy and an Americanized Spencerism (Priego 2012): science was upheld as the key to modernization, yet the elite readily accepted the racist idea—based on U.S.-generated notions of race—that Mexico's large indigenous population was preventing it from evolving into a modern state. Modernity came to be equated with whiteness (Echeverría 2010). The racist view that the majority of Mexico's population was simply too uncivilized to handle liberal democratic governance served as justification for the lengthy Porfirian dictatorship, which went against the tenets of French Liberalism, which had formed the basis of Mexican governance since the 1850s.

In Porfirian logic, Mexico needed science, technology, and liberalism to evolve into a modern society, but it could do so only with the firm hand of the Porfirian state to control its "naturally inferior" and "unruly" indigenous population (Priego 2012). This early history betrays the way Euro-American racism placed the yoke of madness upon Mexico's indigenous people (Horcasitas 2000). Inspired by what is now referred to as scientific racism, Mexican physicians and scientists claimed that through their natural (biological) inferiority, indigenous people were more likely to be both mad and criminal. As Ferguson and Gupta note (2002), there is an important connection between the functioning of modern states and the way they exist in physical space—the construction of the first *manicomios* and the confinement of the mad in the early twentieth century speak to this spatialization (Sacristán 2005). The history of psychiatry in Mexico cannot be separated from the racist legacies of its enduring colonialism.

The Porfiriato ended with the Mexican revolution of 1910, but the Mexican state's concern with modernity and what to do with its indigenous population has persisted (Echeverría 2010). The manicomios of the early twentieth century continued to operate, and although there is no published history of madness in Yucatan, we do know about madness during the Mexican revolutionary state. Ríos Molina's (2009) history of La Castañeda, the General Madhouse of Mexico City, in the first ten years of the revolution, and Guillermo Calderón Narváez's memoirs of life at La Castañeda in the fifteen years before its closing, reflect a preoccupation with science, progress, and modernity. The old Asilo Ayala was part of the same national project that constructed La Castañeda. The institutions weathered the Mexican Revolution and the first half of the twentieth century. Both institutions eventually came to be seen as anachronistic and decrepit and were ultimately closed. When Las Lomas first opened its doors in 1978, it was founded on a promise of modernity. Las Lomas was supposed to counter the frightening images of madness and mental institutions that were pervasive in Mexican society. Its founding—late in the game, nearly ten years after La Castañeda had been closed in the name of progress—was part of an effort to legitimize psychiatry as a scientific entity and to bring Mexican psychiatry into the twentieth century.

What does it mean to be mad in Mexico? Ríos Molina describes the many ways that madness was identified in the early twentieth century: "the mad" included people with mental illness, alcoholics, those suffering from neurosyphilis, dementia, epilepsy, war trauma, and hysteria, gays and lesbians, heroin addicts, marijuana smokers, street brawlers, people suffering from melancholy, and children with intellectual disabilities (2009, 24). Locura, Ríos Molina argues, was not about symptomology; rather, it was about being deemed as deserving of confinement. It was defined by social environment. While madness is not a salient medical term, the concept is useful for thinking through what ultimately leads a patient into the wards of the psychiatric hospital. Who is considered mad today to deserve confinement, just as in the early twentieth century, is determined by a patient's social environment. Just as Río Molina concludes that the internment of a patient at La Castañeda was highly dependent on the family's (in)ability and (un)willingness to care for the patient at home, the internment of patients at Las Lomas also depends on a patient's social and familiar environment.

This is hardly surprising or coincidental. Nearly one hundred years years after the events described in Ríos Molina's book, I observed patients coming to Las Lomas's emergency and outpatient departments time after time, yet I saw admission offered only once, and the offer was declined. Patients came with their family members—spouses, parents, adult children, siblings—who sat in on appointments, offering their own observations, asking questions, and otherwise taking an active role in their family member's care. Most of the time, patients—even those who were very sick—were not admitted because their family was willing to care for them.

The role of family in the psychiatric care and prognosis of people suffering from severe mental illness in Mexico has been recognized by Mexican psychiatrists, who have advocated changing internment policies to allow family to stay with their loved ones in the hospital—an "open door" model described as "ethnopsychiatric" (Villaseñor et al. 2003). Unfortunately, while this model was piloted in a psychiatric hospital in Guadalajara, this approach was never taken at Las Lomas. Instead, family played an integral part of outpatient care, and it appeared that it was only when the caretaking family structure failed that patients were admitted. The importance of family structure in the lives of people with mental illness in Mexico cannot be overstated, although this is not unique: it mirrors risk factors and outcomes of severe mental illness in other countries. Doctors at Las Lomas frequently complained that the hospital was a space of social abandonment: families and local authorities would bring elderly patients suffering from dementia, or village drunks who needed to be kept out of the way, and leave them there.

MODERNITY

Mexico's preoccupation with modernity is visible in many settings, particularly in state and public discourse, where the nation is frequently portrayed as floundering on what appears to be an evolutionary journey toward it (Echeverria 2010). This is visible in the writings of Mexican public intellectuals like Federico Reyes Heroles, Carlos Mayer-Serra, and journalist Jorge Ramos (Reyes Heroles 2015; Ramos 2015; Mayer-Serra 2014). These writers, publishing in large-circulation national newspapers such as *Excelsior* and *El País*, frequently depict modernity as a destination, usually as they criticize the government for thwarting the journey. For instance, in response to a controversial statement made by President Enrique Peña Nieto that Mexico was plagued by a culture of corruption, Carlos Mayer-Serra decried, "If we accept that corruption is cultural, *we would have to accept that the modernization of our country is not possible in the short term*" (2014; emphasis mine). Mayer-Serra's assertion reflects an ongoing anxiety about the project of modernization in Mexico. Writing about the challenges of modernity in Yucatan, historian Gilbert Joseph (2010) observes that Mexico's leaders have long been preoccupied with modernity: "Since independence, at least, Mexico's leaders have shown themselves doggedly determined to pursue the chimera of 'modernity,' whether defined by liberal, positivist, revolutionary, or neoliberal politicians and technocrats of the state, or by modernizing agents of the Catholic Church. More often than not, these would-be engineers have found themselves frustrated by stubborn Mexican realities" (274).

The anxiety expressed in Mexico's public discourse on modernity was also articulated by many of my urban-dwelling, middle-class interlocutors, especially those who were medical providers. One day, I arrived at the acute ward at Las Lomas a little early. The attending psychiatrist had not arrived, but one of her residents, Maria Luisa, a first-year resident from Guadalajara, Mexico's second largest city, was there. Maria Luisa and I had not had an opportunity to get to know each other very well, but she knew who I was, and she was eager to hear more about my research. I asked her, as we chatted, what she thought about Las Lomas and Yucatan generally.

She made a face. "Honestly, what really bothers me about this state is that people have no culture."

This was a familiar complaint, the kind of complaint that *huaches* (a hispanized version of *Huach* [*waach*], a Yucatec Maya word meaning "foreigner" typically used by Maya and non-Maya speakers alike to describe a Mexican who is not from Yucatan, but most frequently from Central Mexico or Mexico City) make when they come Yucatan. I tried to maintain a passive expression, although as an anthropologist and as a Yucatecan, I found the statement off-putting.

"What do you mean?" I asked.

She shrugged. "Well, these people, the local population, they don't stand up for themselves. They just let the government walk all over them. They don't *know* what their rights are! They aren't aware of their rights, they're completely ignorant. There is no culture of civic engagement. That's not what it's like at all in Guadalajara. There, people know their rights, they demand their rights be respected. If the government does something they don't like, they mobilize, take to the streets to demonstrate."

Maria Luisa did not use the words "modern," or "modernity," but this brief conversation reflected her beliefs about citizenship, rights, and civic engagement. For Maria Luisa, to "have culture" meant being an informed, engaged citizen willing to hold one's government accountable. Her words imply a modern, neoliberal subject. In her work among mental health care providers in Oaxaca, another Mexican state with a large population of indigenous people that, like Yucatan, is often stereotyped as backward and "not modern," Whitney Duncan (2017) identifies a similar discourse blaming local culture as an obstacle to modernization.

While Maria Luisa does not view "culture" as an obstacle of modernization, but rather defines it by its absence, the difference between her statement and those of Duncan's informants is superficial and predicated on two different understandings of the word. For Duncan's informants, "culture" is a collection of "other" things: indigenous language, "magical thinking," localized customs and beliefs incongruent with the self-actualized, rational subject valued by the current mental health care model. For Maria Luisa, the fact that people in Yucatan are not following her idea of an informed (hence, rational and self-actualized) citizenry implies an *absence* of culture because in her eyes, "culture" is inherently modern and Western—the concept of culture most of us try to dispel when we teach introductory anthropology courses—and any variation from this concept is "not-culture." Both discourses value a vision of modernity situated in the Global North and devalue any worldview that does not embrace it.

If rationality is the hallmark of the modern neoliberal subject (Rose 1996), madness is its foil. In his classic history of madness and modernity, Foucault (1988a) portrays a story of "insanity in an age of reason"—the existence of madness and the mad in daily life gave way to their gradual exclusion of society. But with the emergence of modern states and the driving logics of biopolitics and biopower comes an interest in rehabilitation and the "psy sciences" (Rose 1996). In Rose's history, the psy sciences were a pivotal part of the emergence of the neoliberal subject. They function to help modern states first understand, then control, the behaviors of their populations. The neoliberal individual emerges as a self-aware, rational actor, the strongest ally in maintaining the functionality of the modern state. The challenge of madness to modernity lies in its inherent irrationality. Moreover, the narratives of Foucault's *Madness and Civilization* (1988) and Rose's *Inventing Ourselves* (1996), as enticing as they are, find challenges in the ethnographic contexts in which I and others work (Jenkins 2015). Where anthropologists have, in Jenkins's words, "become enamored of Foucault's biopolitics and technologies of the self," many of us working in the Global South (or the Global Middle, as I tend to think of Mexico) find that the local—notions of self, experiences of psychiatric disease, social organization—complicates narratives of modernity and rationality put forth by Foucault and Rose.

In the context of Latin America, this complication was acknowledged in the writings of one from its own intelligentsia: Argentinian anthropologist Nestor García Canclini, reflecting on what he calls "Latin American contradictions," notes the region has had "an exuberant modernism alongside a deficient modernization" (1989, 65); in other words, Mexico and Latin America can be understood as societies that have modernism without modernization. Another way to understand this is by considering Mignolo's (2011) assertion: "'Modernity' is a complex narrative whose point of origination was Europe; a narrative that builds Western civilization by celebrating its achievement while hiding at the same time its darker side, 'coloniality.' Coloniality, in other words, is constitutive of modernity—there is no modernity without coloniality" (3).

Without using the language of coloniality, García Canclini (1989, 2005) makes a similar argument. Like Octavio Paz before him, he considers the role played by Latin America's former colonizers in the formation of the contemporary Mexican state. He characterizes Spain as the "most backward" of European nations. Because Spain was long subject to the Counter-Reformation and other antimodern movements, it was only after independence in the nineteenth century that the new nations could take on the serious projects of modernity. In Mexico, the decision to embrace nineteenth-century classical liberal values associated with modernity—democratic rule, secularism, and industrialization—came about only after the *Guerra de Reforma* (War of Reform, 1858–1861) and a period of French intervention (1861–1867). Mexican modernity, García Canclini laments, is incomplete for a simple reason: the limited democratization of its people. By limiting access to quality schooling, the Mexican elite were able to maintain the status quo without what Foucault and Rose (but notably, not García Canclini) would call a population of self-aware, self-regulating modern subjects. Mexico has experienced several "modernizing moments," such as Benito Juarez's 1857 constitution (which effectively made Mexico a secular state), the embrace in Porfirian Mexico of science and technology, the 1917 adoption of the most progressive constitution of its time, and the Mexican Renaissance, an artistic revolution led by the likes of Diego Rivera, José Clemente Orozco, David Alfaro Siqueiros, and Frida Kahlo in the aftermath of the revolution. However, these moments stand in sharp contrast to the persistently colonial social structure of Mexican society.

For García Canclini, Latin American modernity can only be understood as a product of a hybrid history. It cannot look like the modern ideals of progress, science, and technology prevalent in the Global North. Of course, modernity everywhere, including in the Global North, is not comprised of self-actualized neoliberal subjects going about their lives, embodying the ideals instilled upon them by the logics of biopower and governmentality. Reality everywhere is more complex. Garcia Canclini argues those artifacts we typically think of as "culture"—art (tourist and otherwise) and music, the ultimate expressions of subjectivity—showcase the inevitable hybridity of modernity, the inevitable way local and global, "modern" and "traditional" encounter and transform each other in unexpected ways.

García Canclini's hybridity—much like Mignolo's coloniality—is useful for thinking through the complexity of Yucatecan indigeneity, but only if read alongside its critics. One of the most salient critiques of García Canclini's hybridity is that the discourse of hybridity presents an essentialist interpretation of indigenous people and experiences (Rivera Cusicanqui 2012, 100). Hybridity is too close to homogenization and *mestizaje*, the general process of mixing indigenous, African, and Spanish ancestries (to be revisited in more detail in chapter 2), concepts that erase indigenous experience and gloss over the foundational violence of the colonial encounter. In his introduction to the English translation of *Culturas Híbridas*, García Canclini (2005, xxiv) notes that his concept of hybridization leaves room for contradiction and shies away from homogenizing discourses. In this vein, hybridization is a flexible, open-ended concept. The inherent contradiction—and internalized conflict—of hybridity, he argues, makes it useful for thinking through Latin American modernity and, I would add, for understanding the ways in which Latin American modernity is inherently colonial.

Over and over, in my research and that of others, the Mexican state's obsession with becoming *modern* figures prominently. In the late nineteenth and first decade of the twentieth century, during Porfirio Diaz's dictatorship, French positivism came to characterize Mexican architecture, philosophy, and science. Diaz's predecessor, Benito Juarez, was an enlightenment man who embraced the separation of church and state, civil marriage, and human rights. Diaz and Juarez both embraced a dream of a modern Mexico; it was a dream that reverberated in a different form through the Mexican revolution and what eventually became a gradual de-revolution, as the principles of the 1917 constitution were betrayed, article by article, with the privatization of resources previously said to belong to the Mexican people—in other words, to no one (Breglia 2006). Now, rather than belonging to no one, these resources belong to Mexican elites, foreign expats, and transnational corporations.

The public intellectuals who publish in Mexican papers and online sources in the twenty-first century continue to write about how far the Mexican state continues to be from this utopian vision of modernity, even as García Canclini proposed that Mexico, a "hybrid culture," should find its own way in—and out of—modernity. I do not share this optimism, in part because I agree with Walter Mignolo's assertion that coloniality is the darker side of Western modernity, and modernity as we know it cannot exist without coloniality. Coloniality, an inherently oppressive mode of existence, persists in Mexico more than 200 years after independence, and almost 100 years to the date from the adoption of what was considered the most progressive, revolutionary constitution of its time: the 1917 constitution, a manifestation of Mexico's modern dream.[4]

Although what modernity looks like has shifted over time, most would agree that in the twentieth and twenty-first centuries, modernity looks like a prosperous nation: peaceful streets, a healthy GDP, no corruption, a robust and constantly updated infrastructure, thriving science and technology sectors, and a healthy population, among other measures. With the failure of previous economic models characterized by protectionism and Import-Substitution-Industrialization in the twentieth century (Levy-Orlick 2009), the adoption of the North American

Free Trade Agreement (NAFTA) signaled the embrace of what has become the neoliberal world order: the transnational takeover of the Mexican economy.[5] Science, technology, and unbridled capitalism have fully integrated Mexico into the global economy. This is irreversible. And yet, as all of this has happened, there is a national sentiment of disgust with the country's government. Accusations of cronyism and corruption are leveled at both major national political parties, Partido Revolucionario Institucional (PRI) and Partido de Acción Nacional (PAN). In the end, the two parties seem to differ only in the faces of those who benefit from their policies, not in their substance.

Las Lomas stands at the threshold of modernity. By this, I do not mean that the hospital is in a transition from some sort of revolutionary pseudosocialist system toward a neoliberal modality of existence, as if this progression were smooth or unidirectional. This would presuppose the existence of a revolutionary pseudosocialist system and neoliberal modality of existence as separate, coherent stages in an evolutionary time line. As I will demonstrate in this book, there is no time line, and these seemingly defined "stages" are, in fact, messy, largely dysfunctional abstractions sharing a persistent, unshakeable strain of colonialism. What I mean is that Las Lomas occupies a space "between": between sanity and madness, between modernity and anachronism. This "medieval dungeon" now stands, as the old Asilo Ayala and La Castañeda once did, as everything that was wrong with the old vision of modernity. Soon, it will be out with the old once again, but what the future holds remains unknown.

COLONIALITY

"Coloniality," a term coined by Aníbal Quijano (1992), describes the continuation of colonial relationships beyond colonization, an idea previously articulated as "internal colonialism" by Mexican sociologist Pedro González Casanova (1969). This term describes the way Mexico and other former colonies, despite winning independence from Spain in 1821, continue to maintain a colonial relationship with their own peoples through regional elites, who are mostly descendants of the European colonizers, while they exploit the labor and resources of the indigenous and indigenous-descended majority. Coloniality exists on a global scale in what Quijano (2000) calls the "colonial matrix of power," a materialist model that sees coloniality as largely tied to political economy. Neoliberalism, as an economic development strategy, is merely the current iteration of the colonial matrix of power. In Mexico, coloniality is visible beyond economic models, partially achieved through a cultural valuing of Western modernity and an accompanying, persistent racism. At the same time elites continue to maintain a colonial relationship with the lower classes, the Mexican state also continues to occupy a subservient geopolitical position vulnerable to global economic changes and heavily reliant, because of neoliberal economic policy, on an essentially colonial, if troubled, relationship with the United States.

Quijano's coloniality presents the role of racism as the foundational principle of colonial and postcolonial political economy. It refers to the way race—conceptualized as European versus non-European—intersects with capital to produce various forms of hierarchical labor (forced, coercive, reciprocal, salaried, and so forth). The notion that the colonial order was founded on racism was articulated by Frantz Fanon ([1961] 2004, [1952] 2008) and has been further developed by other scholars of coloniality such as Silvia Rivera Cusicanqui (2012), Ramón Grosfoguel (2011b), Boaventura de Sousa Santos (2010), and Walter Mignolo (2011). Fanon, a black Martinican psychiatrist writing about the Algerian struggle against French colonialism, is a natural ally, but a problematic one: Fanon's *Wretched of the Earth*, a book I turn to because of his engagement with the effects of colonialism on the native psyche, was published in 1961. His context is a much more modern colonialism than the one that exists in Mexico. By the time the Fanon wrote about Algerians rising up against the French colonial order, Mexico had already gone through a revolution that predated the one in Russia, survived its violent aftershocks, carried out a massive project of land reform, and expropriated its oil from foreign investors. In 1961, the Mexican state was still seven years away from massacring "30–300" students at the Plaza de las Tres Culturas in Tlatelolco.

All these events—the revolution, agrarian reform, the expropriation of oil, the massacre at Tlatelolco—are directly relevant to Las Lomas today. These events form part of Mexican national memory, created or managed deliberately and systematically by the Mexican state. They are also part of local collective memory, even in the backwaters of Yucatan, where Lázaro Cardenas first carried out the experiment that would be known as *la reforma agraria*, the experiment whose end inspired the Zapatista movement in another Mayan region, Chiapas. In Yucatan, this collective memory is identified in what rural inhabitants refer to as the *época de la esclavitud*, the time of slavery. Like others (Castañeda 1996; Breglia 2006; Fallaw 2001), I encountered this collective memory of *esclavitud* over my years of fieldwork in various regions of the state. The memory does not refer to the Spanish colonial period or to a lasting memory of European subjugation, but it is more recent; it refers to the time immediately preceding the arrival of Lázaro Cárdenas's agrarian reform in 1935.

Yucatan has been described as "the place the revolution never arrived" (Fallaw 2001). Its economy was heavily reliant on henequen (*Agave fourcroydes Lem*) monoculture. A few wealthy families controlled vast swaths of land dedicated to henequen production, farmed by a mass of destitute workers kept in check by an oppressive system of debt peonage. The eastern region of the peninsula, in contrast, did not depend on henequen in the same way and maintained some balance of independence in large part due to the legacy of the Caste War of the nineteenth century.[6]

The commonly accepted narrative is that President Lázaro Cárdenas (1934–1940) chose Yucatan as an experimental site for his agrarian reform program precisely because the oppressive conditions of the debt-peonage system would ensure support from the peasantry. Cárdenas appropriated and redistributed some 180,000 km² to peasants throughout Mexico, establishing the *ejido* system of communally owned land under Article 27 of the 1916 constitution. While historian Ben Fallaw (2001) argues that Cárdenas's top-down approach, which left little room for local agency, undermined his iconic program, people in Yucatan today continue to remember the hardship of esclavitud and the sudden redistribution of land as a transformative moment in recent history. This memory of dispossession and repossession holds far more significance for the local population today than does the monumental architecture of the Ancient Maya (Castañeda 1996; Breglia 2006).

Esclavitud itself never came up at Las Lomas. Esclavitud always seemed to appear in quiet afternoons in the countryside, in places like Yaxche', a village of 400 located thirty kilometers south of the ancient ruins of Uxmal. We—my friends and I—might be sitting on doorsteps, watching kids ride by on their bicycles or the neighbor walking down the road to the *Rosario*—a communal reciting of a rosary, a common social activity in Yucatecan villages. In May the days are hot and dry, but when the sun begins to set, the breeze comes in and while the house is stifling, there is nothing like sitting on the front stoop, eating *chico sapote* (*manilkara zapota*), a sweet fruit with a brown peel and a light orange flesh, off the tree. We sit and eat and chat, and the dryness makes the air smell like dust. But it is okay, because we know the rains will come in June, and soon enough the daily rain will cool things down as we go into the summer. In such moments of leisure is when stories of esclavitud come out. In my experience, stories of esclavitud were shared when a curious child—or sometimes, a clueless anthropologist in the field for the first time—asked questions about the past, something as innocent as "What did you do before there was a mill in Yaxche'?"

"Well, in the time of slavery," my friend Candelaria might say, eating her sapote, "the *uchbeen maako'ob* [the old ones][7] had to use a stone mortar and pestle. That was before we had mills. My grandmother said it would take her four hours to grind enough corn for the day's tortillas, oof!"—she'd throw the pit on the gravel road in front of us—"that was hard work, back then."

One day, I pressed on about this time of slavery. "Who were the people slaves to?"

"Oh, I don't know. A family from Merida. They are long gone. They still own the structures in the next village over, the crumbling chimney and the hacienda church with the roof that caved in. But I've never seen them. I don't even know their names."

Another day, I asked if there was anyone alive who remembered the days of slavery. "Old *Mamá Concha*," Candelaria said, referring to her nonagenarian grandmother, "she remembers times of war when she was a child. They had to run and hide in caves from time to time. She remembers when the train station still functioned and there was no road. People didn't take a road to the next town over, they took the train."

Mamá Concha was ninety-four in 2003, when this conversation took place. She was born in 1908, two years before the revolution, and was in her late twenties when Cardenas's land reform came to Yucatan. By the time I mastered enough Maya to chat with her, Mamá Concha had developed dementia, and I was unable to have a conversation with her about her experiences of the past. She passed away in 2009. But her stories of esclavitud, like those of others of her generation, are still told in Yaxche'. They make up a collective memory that informs the lives of those who benefited from agrarian reform and their descendants. This memory of slavery is thus not tied to the experience of European colonialism, but it is connected through its relationship to subjugation, dispossession, and oppression; it is a colonial experience.

For Fanon, colonialism acts directly on the body and psyche of the colonial subject. For the colonized subject, Fanon says, to live is merely to not die—a condition that finds an echo in Agamben's description of bare life. Colonialism is a "systematized negation of the other, a frenzied determination to deny the other any attribute of humanity" (Fanon 1961, 182). The oppressive conditions of colonialism are such that colonial subjects are reduced to simply existing. In its symbolic and actual brutality, the colonial regime wears on the colonized subjects' psyche. When one picks up *The Wretched of the Earth* more than fifty years after its publication, one is struck by its continued timeliness, particularly when it comes to Fanon's vivid descriptions of the impact of colonial violence on the colonized psyche, or what Homi Bhabha (2004) calls the psycho-affective experience of the colonized subject.

By the same token, one is also struck by Fanon's optimism. What book would he have written had he lived to see the results of decolonization? His argument would have probably centered on the incomplete nature of decolonization— former colonies everywhere continue to be subject to the whims and power of their former colonizers. In the era of globalization, hegemonic states continue to lose power to transnational corporations, yet the balance of power continues to lie in the Global North. Coloniality, even after colonialism, is alive and well. Mignolo's assertion that modernity cannot exist without the repressive intricacies of the colonial system returns to haunt. In Yucatan, where decolonization allegedly happened not once, but twice (once in 1821, and once in 1935), the facts seem to bear this out. Is Fanon's colonized subject the same in Algeria as it is in Yucatan? Mignolo argues that without coloniality, modernity is impossible. Coloniality is "the darker side of modernity," inherent to its very existence (2011, 2).

The answer, he proposes, is the "decolonial" option, not a nationalistic entrench-ment as Fanon had hoped for and imagined fifty years prior, but a reinterpreta-tion of the future and a turn to the left. For Mignolo, the Zapatistas in Chiapas stand as an example of a decolonial future.

Is this a decolonial book? Practically, no. In my work at Las Lomas and my years of research in Mexico, I find it difficult to share Mignolo's optimism about deco-lonial alternatives to modernity. A decolonizing book would have a more applied or activist bend. In this book I do little more than show the internal machinery of a state institution in a slice in time. Yet at the same time, this "slice" reveals how the dysfunction that has marked the Mexican state since it was first conceived per-meates the very psyche of its inhabitants. If anything, in this book I reveal the inherent dysfunction of modern neocolonial states through a Mexican case study. The Global North maintains its world dominance because of the dysfunction of places like Mexico.

Is this a decolonial book? Epistemologically, yes. By engaging with the works of indigenous anthropologists like Audra Simpson (2007, 2014) and Joseph Gone (2014) in addressing questions of ethnographic entrapment in chapter 2, by con-versing with Ramón Grosfoguel (2011a, 2011b), Silvia Rivera Cusicanqui (2010, 2012), and Juan Castillo Cocom's (2005) visions of coloniality and modernity throughout this text, by writing from a perspective that is epistemologically grounded in Fanon's work, I engage in deliberate epistemic decolonization, not merely for its own sake, but because these works best highlight the inherent colo-niality of Las Lomas and contemporary Mexican medical care.

My core goal in this book is to demonstrate how the treatment and experience of madness in Mexico are produced by the inherent coloniality of the postrevo-lutionary state. To achieve this goal, it is necessary to approach this complex web of social structure and social relations in an intersectional way—not only in the sense of intersectional feminism but also by attending to the intersections of large- and small-scale levels of social structure. In the same way that Google Earth zeros in on a location, this book first approaches broader questions of indigene-ity and the place of indigenous people in Mexican and Yucatecan society, then gradually moves into the Mexican health care system and the wards of Las Lomas, exploring the inside of the institution, the interactions between doctors and patients, and finally, the intersubjective, lived experiences of the patients them-selves. These experiences constitute the end point of a large and complex neoco-lonial bureaucracy that deserves as much attention as the patients themselves.

MENTAL ILLNESS IN MEXICO

The Mexican Department of Health estimates the prevalence of mental illness in Mexico at between 19 and 24 percent of the population, a percentage compara-ble with that of the United States (World Health Organization 2017). However, while the United States has 16 psychiatrists per 100,000 people, Mexico has 2.7. This means that only 2.5 percent of those suffering from mental illness are ever treated within the mental health care system—although, as I will later describe, there is a robust network of locally available traditional medical practitioners that can and do succeed in treating mental illness. But despite what is considered an abysmal availability of mental health providers, the picture of severe mental illness in Yucatan and Mexico is more complex than it may initially seem. The example of schizophrenia, one of the most documented mental illnesses in the world, illustrates this point.

Longitudinal studies of schizophrenia demonstrate this most devastating of psychiatric ailments has a better course of illness in the Global South than it does in the Global North (Luhrmann and Marrow 2016). Patients in the Global South, on average, tend to see an improvement in their symptoms over time and lose fewer years of healthy life because of their ailment. The disease burden for schizophrenia in Mexico mirrors this trend. A commonly used measure of disease burden is the Disability-Adjusted Life Year, or DALY. DALY is an estimate of years of healthy life lost due to illness or disability, and it is frequently used as a comparative way of understanding the impact of mental illness. While the estimated annual years of healthy life lost due to schizophrenia for people in the United States stands at 258.9 per 100,000 people, and at 263.3 per 100,000 people in Canada (the highest in the continent), Mexico's estimated years of healthy life lost due to schizophrenia falls close to the lower middle in Latin America at 185.8 per 100,000 people (HealthGrove 2013). People who suffer from schizophrenia in Mexico therefore do not have the same bleak outlook that people in the United States and Canada have, although the outlook is worse than Guatemala (137.7) and Haiti (159.7), the two countries with the lowest years of healthy life lost due to schizophrenia that also, ironically, happen to be the poorest.

Although there is no consensus on why the course of illness for schizophrenia in the Global South appears to be better than in the Global North, anthropologist Byron Good (1997) identifies four factors to explain this phenomenon: local interpretations of mental illness, presence of extended family, forms of labor available for the sick person to engage in, and basic social environment. If one imagines these hypotheses as intersecting factors, Mexico's place in the middle of the disease burden reflects its place in the "Global Middle," as a nation that, although still facing major challenges and obstacles, maintains the second-strongest economy of Latin America, a flawed but robust social safety net (primarily in the form of universal access to health care), and free and compulsory primary and secondary (K–9) education. Three of the factors identified by Byron Good—local interpretations of mental illness, forms of labor available, and basic social environment—vary widely throughout the territory and across social classes.

As I have written elsewhere (Reyes-Foster 2013a, 2016a), local etiologies of mental illness coexist with biomedical approaches in Yucatan. Within the state, local interpretations of mental illness vary. For many, particularly people who inhabit rural communities, understandings of mental illness are intimately tied to notions of the person. As Hirose (2008) and I (Reyes-Foster 2013a) have described, for many in Yucatan, particularly those whom anthropologists and others refer to as "Maya," the person is understood as an unbounded self, extending outside the body and into physical space. The individual self is comprised of body, two different types of spirit (*pixan*, the individual immortal soul, and *ool*, a mortal life force inhabiting the blood), and *iknal*, which is best described as a sort of physical presence that remains in highly frequented places, even in the absence of the physical body (Castillo Cocom et al. 2017; Reyes-Foster 2016b; Rodriguez and Castillo Cocom 2010; Hanks 1990). Illness occurs when something goes wrong with any one of those elements, and the balance delicately maintained between these components is upset.

People in these communities who become ill make use of the multiple medical systems available to them. While they will use locally available public medical care—most communities will have a *promotora de salud* (a community health worker), a *pasante* (a recently graduated medical doctor completing her required year of social service), a local publicly funded *centro de salud* (health clinic, or, in larger towns and small cities, a hospital)—they will also readily make use of traditional medical practitioners such as *yerbateros* (herbal specialists), *hueseros* (bone-setters and massage specialists), and *jmeeno'ob* (religious specialists with a wide range of skills and in-depth knowledge of the healing properties of plants). When someone first becomes unwell—for instance, a woman who suffers from *nervios*[8] and begins to have trouble sleeping, experiences intrusive negative memories from her past, and finds herself unusually irritable and prone to flying into a fit of anger—she will go to the most convenient practitioner available, and then will likely visit another if she does not experience an immediate improvement. She will visit her local centro de salud, where the doctor will likely prescribe her a benzodiazepine. She may also visit the local jmeen, who might perform a *santiguar* (a spiritual cleanse), to clear her spirit of bad winds. This woman will not see any contradiction between going to the centro de salud and visiting the jmeen, affirming her belief that both medical systems work in their own way.

Although making use of multiple medical systems is common practice for all kinds of illnesses, mental illness lends itself particularly well to highly localized interpretation. Local etiologies of health tend to construct symptoms commonly understood as being linked to mental health—sleep disturbances, manic states, visual or auditory hallucinations—as spiritual afflictions. These symptoms are commonly explained as the result of unknowingly becoming exposed to a bad wind, or even, in some cases, to demonic intervention. Human activity without proper ritual—making *milpa* without making offerings to the *Aluxo'ob* (trickster dwarves who inhabit the rural landscape), overhunting the deer population, killing a sacred animal without permission—can invite this external intervention from spirits, winds, and demons. For example, in a village I visited in 2008, Xulab, the suicides of two adolescent girls within one month of each other were explained by some of the villagers as a sign that the town needed a sacred "tying" ritual, a *loj kaaj tal*, to keep the forest spirits out of the town perimeter. When I pressed them further, asking how the villagers knew this was the case, they explained that a deer had been spotted in the village square shortly before the first suicide and a badger before the second. The entrance of wildlife into spaces conceived as domesticated was seen as a bad omen, a belief I have heard expressed in other Yucatecan villages. In Xulab, people believed the young girls had fallen prey to demonic intervention. When Lidia, the local *promotora de salud* (community health technician) began to suffer from nightmares and intrusive thinking, she, too, understood her symptoms as having a demonic etiology. Lidia explained that a combination of therapy, medication, and prayer had restored her health.

Elsewhere (Reyes-Foster 2013a, 2016a), I have argued that in Yucatan, biomedical models of care easily comingle with traditional medicine, although biomedical practitioners and institutions are, on the whole, hostile to traditional medical models of care. As Yucatec Maya medical anthropologist Miguel Güemez Pineda once said to me, what is remarkable about mental illness in Yucatan is the fact that the vast majority of the state's mentally ill never need to be committed to Las Lomas. Between the jmeeno'ob and the local clinic, most people who suffer from mental health problems, even severe illness, are able to live their lives without contact with the institution. If a patient becomes sick enough that involuntary treatment becomes necessary, it is likely that the patient and their family have exhausted all other means of care.

Involuntary commitment frequently appears to be the result of a failure in a patient's immediate circle, most often in their immediate family. While Eva's story will be revisited later in this book, here I emphasize that her family's dysfunction played a central role in her illness. Her mother's legal troubles and the fact that she was already the primary caretaker of a severely disabled child meant that she was unable to take on the burden of caring for Eva when she became ill. When Eva's mother, a woman in her sixties with a friendly face and a kind smile, met Eva's attending psychiatrist, Dr. Tun, she expressed her regret at Eva's hospitalization: "If I had known, *doctora*. If I had known and if I had time. I would have come and stayed in her apartment with her. Made sure she was eating, sleeping. Made sure she got off to work every day. Gotten her in to see a doctor before things became this bad! We all want her to succeed, you see. I could have gotten her through this. But I'm so busy. I have little Javier to look after and then this problem with my son-in-law. . . ."

Eva's mother describes what is locally recognized as the appropriate way to behave when one's child is ill: visit, stay, and ensure the child has adequate rest, nutrition, and medical care. Dr. Tun agreed that Eva would likely not have needed hospitalization if a family member had been with her and noticed her symptoms when they first appeared. It was her isolation, Dr. Tun concluded, that allowed Eva's health to spiral out of control so quickly. Although this may have been the case, both Dr. Tun's assessment and Eva's mother's statements betray a set of beliefs about the role of family in times of distress, a set of beliefs that is also apparent in J. R.'s admonition to Juan Vasquez: "I would sooner lock a relative of mine in a room in my house before I would ever bring him to your 'hospital,'" J. R. wrote, betraying the belief that family is ultimately responsible for caring for their afflicted kin.

Eva's story also illustrates the diversity and variability of life in contemporary Yucatan. There are many people, like Lidia, the community health technician from Xulab, who reside in agricultural communities and rarely ever leave them, but there are many others, like Eva, who travel throughout the state in search of work or an education (Castañeda 1996; Re Cruz 1996; Breglia 2006). Whenever possible, they commute back and forth between their hometowns and their places of employment or school. Sometimes, however, commuting is impossible, and staying with relatives may be considered the best option. By living alone, Eva was breaking with tradition—most Yucatecans live with family until they marry—but she is part of a small but growing number of young people who are opting to live independently.

Thus, the strength and cohesion of the family unit in Yucatan, as in other places, appears to have a protective element when it comes to the course of severe mental illness. While I encountered patients from all walks of life at Las Lomas, what many of the sickest patients seemed to share was familial isolation arising from difficulty of some kind within the family: marital strife, conflict with stepfamily, or estrangement. I am not arguing that this isolation caused or affected the course of their mental illness, but I do see it as an important factor in their involuntary commitment. As I discuss in chapter 3, lack of a familial support network is a major factor in cases of abandonment, and it has been identified as a major problem across Mexican psychiatric institutions by Disability Rights International (2011).

THE SETTING

Las Lomas, when seen from the outside, mirrors its crumbling interior. It sits within what used to be the outer perimeter of Merida, the largest metropolitan area in the state (population about one million), and it has steadily been swallowed up by the expanding city. A poorly maintained, occasionally painted, squat, one-story structure is the entrance to what is actually a relatively large campus of several different poorly maintained, squat, one-story structures housing various wards, offices, and medical examination rooms. The 139-bed facility provides in- and outpatient services to about 70,000 people each year. In 2008, the facility housed a psychiatric emergency room, an acute ward, a long-term care ward, and outpatient consultation offices. In addition, the hospital housed electro-convulsive therapy (ECT) equipment, an outpatient pediatric wing, classroom spaces, a kitchen and seating area, a pharmacy, medical records department, and administrative offices for its medical, psychological, social work, nursing, and support personnel. When I returned in 2012, an additional building with a separate entrance, which housed more outpatient psychological care services like individual and group therapy, had been constructed. The hospital had fifty-eight full-time employees, including support staff, social workers, psychologists, and psychiatrists. Las Lomas is also a teaching hospital, providing training to local medical students, hosting twelve psychiatry and six integrative medicine residents who arrive from all over Mexico to complete their specializations, and serving as a practicum site for students completing studies in psychology, nursing, and social work.

The foundational data for this book come from three different research periods in Yucatan: twelve months in 2008 as part of dissertation fieldwork on suicide and suicide prevention, three months in 2012, and another two months in 2013. In addition to these primary research periods, I have been actively engaged in the region as a field researcher since 2003, when I conducted my first independent field research project. I carried out preliminary research and Yucatec Mayan language training in 2005, 2006, and 2007. My research sites have not been limited to Las Lomas or even the Merida metropolitan area, although the Las Lomas facility is the primary setting of this book: over the years, I have spent extended periods of time in Valladolid, a small city (population about 70,0000) about 159 kilometers from the capital city of Merida and its surrounding villages, and in a village I call Yaxche', located near the municipality of Muna in the former henequen-producing region of southern Yucatan.

The data that support this book comprise hundreds of pages of handwritten field notes taken in 2008 and 2012 inside Las Lomas and ninety-seven electronic field notes collected in 2012 and 2013. These notes include daily field observations, notes taken during observations of group and individual treatment sessions, case presentations, and everyday interactions, and notes taken during informal and formal interviews. In 2008, I spent three full days a week at Las Lomas, attending regular meetings, therapy sessions, and other activities in the suicide prevention program, *La Esperanza*. In 2012 alone, I witnessed over 200 medical interactions and spent four to five days a week at Las Lomas, rotating between the acute ward, the emergency room, and three outpatient consultation practices. Between 2008 and 2013, I collected approximately sixty interviews from patients, family members, psychologists, psychiatrists, and volunteers. Although I concluded primary fieldwork in 2013, since then I have made nearly annual visits to Merida and maintained close ties with former interlocutors, particularly the people I call Juan Vasquez and Maria Tun. I last visited Las Lomas in July 2016, when I was given a tour of the facility after significant renovations were made.

A brief comment on my own positionality within this research is warranted here. I was born in Merida and spent part of my early childhood there before emigrating to the United States, where I have lived off and on since I was eight years old. I was educated in the United States and grew up in a bicultural, bilingual home. My father, a *yucateco* from Izamal, stayed behind, along with most of my extended family. My mother is what is (not kindly) referred to as a *huach* (a Mexican foreigner in Yucatan); she is from Monterrey, a major city in Northern Mexico just 227 kilometers south of Laredo, Texas. In Yucatecan society, this makes me a *yucahuach*, a child of a Yucatecan and a *huach*. My U.S. upbringing makes me even *more* foreign: *yucateca*, *huach*, and *gringa*, or, as one friend jokingly coined it, a *yuca-huachgringa*. These local identity categories—huach, yucateca, gringa—came together as my interlocutors tried to make sense of me: I dress informally, like a gringa, and I wear comfortable—that is, unstylish—shoes. I do not wear makeup. I am a native Spanish speaker, and when I am in Yucatan long enough, my Yucatecan accent does not let me down. But I write and usually think in English, and I have been accused of having a foreign accent when I speak Spanish. This affects how others view me: I do not fit the trappings of the local middle class or its ideals of femininity. This affects how I view myself: *no soy de aquí, ni soy de allá, pero soy más de allá que de acá.* I am from neither here nor there, but I am more from there (the United States) than I am from here. In this sense, I am a "halfie anthropologist" (Abu-Lughod 1991), conducting research in a culture I understand as a native yet to which I do not fully belong. During more than fifteen years of research in Yucatan, I have found this positionality to be very advantageous, as I am able to present myself as an insider or an outsider depending on particular circumstances.

There are several ways in which my position in local society presents limitations to my study. My appearance clearly marks my racial privilege: as a Mexican immigrant of racially mixed heritage, I grew up hearing that I "didn't *look* Mexican," meaning, of course, that my appearance is more European than it is indigenous. This in and of itself affords me great privilege in Yucatecan society, which—like Mexican society in general—is notoriously racist. It most certainly affected how I was perceived and treated by many of my interlocutors who did not share this privilege. While I have been able to maintain close friendships with many of the people I have encountered in Yucatan over the years, my "white," American privilege is something that I acknowledge and am actively cognizant of in my interactions with interlocutors on the ground.

In addition to my encounters with the inescapable dimensions of race and class, I also met many people who struggled with severe mental illness, psychosis, and suicide attempts. Although I have struggled with anxiety and depression before in my life, I have never been subjected to psychiatric hospitalization or extended psychiatric treatment. I have never experienced psychosis. In this way, the experiences of the patients I interacted with will forever remain, at least on a phenomenological level, alien to me. Furthermore, although I have acquired expertise in mental health, I am not a trained mental health professional, and

I am not a medical doctor. In this sense, the lived experiences of providers also remain alien to me.

ETHICS

What does it mean to do one's research inside the wards of a psychiatric hospital? The question was not as troublesome when I conducted my research in 2008, because my work in the suicide prevention unit was carried out only among people who were capable of providing informed consent. This became an entirely new question when I planned to return to Las Lomas and work in the acute and emergency wards. I looked to my University Institutional Review Board (IRB), expecting obstacles and delays, but when I spoke to the IRB director, she asked only one question: "Are you collecting identifiable information?"

"No," I said. I had never planned to keep identifiable information—names, addresses, phone numbers.

"Okay, then," she smiled brightly, "you should be good. Your project should receive exempt status. Just be clear about that. Is the hospital down there okay with you going? Can they give you a letter of support?"

The answer was yes to both questions. Thus, when I submitted my original research protocol to my university IRB, I clearly stated that I would not collect nor keep identifiable information. I was clear to say that I would be carrying out participant observation research inside the psychiatric hospital, including the acute ward. I provided a letter of support from my sponsor, Juan Vasquez, and I indicated what he told me about Las Lomas's own human subjects research review process: that they had such a process for clinical research, but they did not require one for my particular project, which was in the social sciences.

My project was approved only a few weeks later and granted "exempt" status: the project posed no more than minimal risk and did not need to undergo full board review; the preliminary review was enough. This meant I did not have to collect those infamous informed consent forms; all I had to do was supply my informants with a "study information sheet," which I had already translated into Spanish and supplied to the IRB office. As long as I did not collect identifiable information and obtained clearance from the attending psychiatrists prior to collecting interviews, I was free to do my research at Las Lomas. Meanwhile, Las Lomas itself did not require any additional human subjects review. As surprising as this may seem, I have found other colleagues who have conducted research in clinical settings in Mexico and report similar ease of access. Although Mexico passed the Federal Law for Protection of Personal Data in Possession of Individuals, a law analogous to the Health Insurance Portability and Accountability Act of 1996 (also known as HIPAA, U.S. federal legislation that protects and restricts access to the medical and health information of people using medical services in the United States), I did not find the kind of concern over ethnographic research and patient privacy in Mexican hospitals that I have encountered in U.S. medical institutions. My experience and that of others doing research with vulnerable populations abroad point to a need for further engagement with questions of ethics and the protection of human subjects.

When I arrived at Las Lomas, I experienced a profound sense of unease about conducting research there, particularly in the acute ward. I was welcomed by every doctor I met, and Dr. Maria Tun, attending psychiatrist for the women in the acute ward, took me under her wing. Every day I sat in her consultation room as people were brought in for assessment. Dr. Tun, who deeply enjoyed teaching and mentoring, always had one, usually two, psychiatry or integrative medicine residents working with her during these times. When a patient was brought in for consultation, she could expect to see at least two and up to four people in the room during the evaluation. Dr. Tun would introduce me as an anthropologist after she introduced her residents.

However, many of the patients in the acute ward were experiencing psychosis. They had no idea who I was, or what I was doing there. Although I witnessed what was undoubtedly a private moment, patients did not have an opportunity to decline my presence there anymore than they had an opportunity to decline the presence of the residents who were there to learn. Although I never spoke to patients in these conditions and limited my activities to observing and taking light notes during these interactions, I continued to feel extremely uncomfortable about using any of that material. Having witnessed the treatment of acute psychiatric patients in an underfunded, troubled public institution, using patients' stories that were relayed during what were undoubtedly some of the worst moments of their lives for my own research purposes—without their consent—was unethical, regardless of whether or not I had IRB approval to do it.

Although I collected this data in 2012, I did not begin drafting this manuscript until 2015. There was a time when I did not think I would ever be able to draft it, in large part because while I could not visualize a book that did *not* include the experiences and voices of acute psychiatric patients, I felt deeply uncomfortable using them. When I finally decided that I would write this book, I came to an imperfect solution, but one I felt I could live with. In the first instance, I primarily used materials from patients who *were* able to provide consent. These patients were people who were cleared by their attending physicians and people with whom I conducted one-on-one interviews. With each patient I carried out a consent procedure, during which I explained the purpose of the research and what to expect in our interview, and I assured the patients that they had the ability to decline or withdraw from the study at any time. Twenty-seven acute patients were cleared for interviews by their physicians. Two patients indicated they did not wish to participate in the interview during the consent process, and the interview immediately stopped.

For those patients with whom I interacted only in my role as an observer of the clinical encounter, who were not able to provide informed consent, I faced a different challenge. Rather than merely disguise the identities of these patients, I decided to take elements of their varying experiences and create composite characters as stand-ins. In other words, although all the events, symptoms, and narratives in this book did take place, these composite characters and stories integrate elements from my encounters with several different patients from whom I did not have an opportunity or an ability to obtain consent. I use these composites only in describing patient-physician interactions when the interaction illustrates a key point about the doctor-patient relationship or the experiences of psychiatric patients at Las Lomas, and so generally these composites appear when describing interactions in the acute care ward. This was the only way I felt I could ethically use this material.

THE STRUCTURE OF THIS BOOK

As I outlined earlier in this introduction, madness, modernity, and coloniality are the common threads that hold this book together. In chapter 2, I explore this connection further by examining the creation of "the Maya" as a tourist commodity in Yucatan. Local discourses about "the Maya," constructed as a mysterious people of the ancient past, have produced the figure of Ixtab, a suicide deity, to explain a contemporary phenomenon: a statewide elevated suicide rate. In chapter 2, framing Ixtab within the broader context of the 2012 "Mayan Apocalypse," I present the theoretical foundations of this book. I consider the ways existing frameworks of *mestizaje*, indigenous identity, and class-based discrimination produce colonialist discourses that reify the construct of indigenous people as unstable, while conveniently ignoring the broader psycho-affective effects of coloniality. Building on the work of Fanon ([1961] 2004), Grosfoguel (2011a, 2011b), and de Sousa Santos (2010), I introduce the notion of *Zona del Estar* as a conceptual tool to understand madness and indigeneity from a framework of flexible temporality firmly entrenched in the colonial matrix of power. Madness, suicide, and indigeneity become intertwined in a colonial tangle.

In chapter 3, I describe how the colonial matrix of power is "made" through the interaction of various actors with conflating and competing interests. By exploring the connections between various events inside and outside the ward—cases of abandonment, "cheating" on insurance schemes, and political battles in Las Lomas and other state bureaucracies—I argue that the colonial matrix of power is constituted by a complex web of social processes, producing a contradictory, dysfunctional, and self-propagating system. Clinical encounters reveal much about the construction of Las Lomas as a dysfunctional space as they do about the relationships between patients and providers.

Modernity emerges as a troubling trope in chapter 4, as I present Las Lomas as a strategy and foil in the Mexican state's drive toward modernity. Engaging with notions of the mental institution as asylum and the drive toward independent living as a hallmark of neoliberal subjectivity, I describe the dysfunction that characterizes everyday operations in the hospital. The mission of Las Lomas has always been aligned with values and logics characteristic of Western biomedicine and neoliberal subjectivity—independence, self-actualization, self-care, individual responsibility, and self-sufficiency. But in rhetoric, Las Lomas is no different than any other modern mental institution, as the complexity of Mexico's modernizing project is reflected in the dysfunction of the ward. *Interculturalidad*, a supposedly decolonizing framework that explicitly recognizes the need for linguistic and cultural inclusion in pluricultural Mexico, has become another rhetorically dominant ideology in public health discourse. However, despite a master plan with an explicitly intercultural agenda, the discourse of interculturality has not been accompanied by action. This chapter is an analysis of multiple actors in this ethnographic setting: patients and doctors, but also the institutional and broader structural schema as well. By recalling Walter Mignolo's assertion that coloniality is the darker side of Western modernity, I contend that Las Lomas symbolizes the darker side of Mexican modernity; its dysfunction is rooted in its colonial core, with little hope or sincere desire for change.

In chapter 5, I move away from a grand narrative of social structure and designed sabotage and turn my attention to the everyday enactment of psychiatric care inside Las Lomas. Focusing on medical interactions between doctors and patients, I engage with the notion of madness as a paradox to (rational) liberal individualism. I analyze a series of clinical interactions I recorded over the course of my ethnographic research inside the inpatient and outpatient wards. I consider how patient and doctor interactions coproduce subjectivities grounded in hierarchies of affect and knowledge. These hierarchies coalesce in three ways: through regimes of truth, negotiation, and orientation. For each instance, I present various clinical interactions illustrating how truth, negotiation, and orientation are co-constructed within each encounter. The three regimes are intertwined. "Truth" is the outcome of negotiation in a space produced by physical and symbolic acts of orientation of the clinical encounter.

In chapter 6, I explore the intersubjective experiences of psychiatric patients and their "others" inside the acute ward. Engaging with frameworks of materialism and relationality, I consider the ways in which Fanon's "colonized psyche" can be framed alongside a materialist, ontological analysis of the interactions among patients, invisible beings, and alternative realities in the space of the acute ward. Again, by engaging with the recurrent motifs of modernity and coloniality, I explore in this chapter the lived experiences of patients on the ward.

In my conclusion, the epilogue to this ethnographic account, I return to Las Lomas in 2016, four years after I had completed my research there. I discuss three important shake-ups that had taken place since my 2012 visit: a human rights investigation, a federal takeover, and an employee strike. Each of these events illustrates a progressive and increasingly rapid decline into chaos, a struggle to implement change in an environment that is always changing yet never changes. In the end, Las Lomas is a mirror of the Mexican state, the colonial dark side of Mexican modernity.

2 · COLONIALITY, *LA ZONA DEL ESTAR*, AND YUCATAN'S MAYA HERITAGE

No es possible resistir / de la mestiza el encanto
Pues se conmueve hasta un santo / al ver su terno lucir

It is impossible to resist / the charm of the mestiza
For even a saint would be moved / to see her show off her dress
—Cirilo Baqueiro Preve, "La Mestiza"

Imagine the bustling colonial city of Merida, Yucatan. *La Plaza*, its central square, full of lush, green trees surrounding a flagpole flying the Mexican flag, is surrounded by the largest Spanish colonial cathedral of its time, the imposing architecture of the conquistador's house, and the state government and municipal palaces. The square is full of people: white tourists, brown locals, young girls wearing traditional clothing from Chiapas (a different region of Mexico), and old *mestizas* wearing the Yucatecan *huipil*, a white cotton dress with richly embroidered hem and collar, sitting on wooden milk crates, selling bags of sliced mangoes sprinkled with chili out of plastic tubs. Red double-decker buses take tourists to the parts of town the local guides have found to be popular. The smells of fried plantains, cars, heat, and sweat hang heavy in the air.

If one takes a short stroll from the main square—it has to be very early in the morning or in the evening; at any other time the heat makes the sidewalks and pavement glimmer—one sees the classic signs of a tourist destination: money-exchange shops, boutique hotels for the yuppies, hostels for the hippies, gourmet restaurants and trendy bars for the hipsters and the local elites. But more than everything else, there are the shops, and—to paraphrase Kenny McCormick's description of hell—they all sell the same thing: Maya culture. Maya glyphs and art on vases and tapestries. Ceramic and cement replicas of Maya figurines found in archaeological contexts. Locally and not-so-locally produced textiles. Panama hats. Crystals. Hammocks. Living beetles decorated with rhinestones. All these

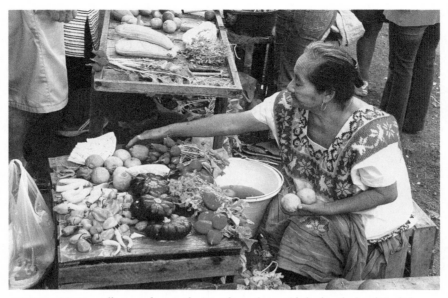

FIGURE 1. Mestiza selling produce in the Merida market, published in the local English-language magazine *Yucatan Today*. Artist: Juan Manuel Mier y Terán Calero. Courtesy of *Yucatan Today*.

items are furtively connected to a construction commonly known as Maya culture, but among them, the figure of the *mestiza*, an indigenous woman wearing the traditional huipil, stands out.

La mestiza is the epitome of Yucatecan Maya-ness. Inside the local restaurants of *centro*, mestizas in huipiles sit around fake hearths, *torteando*—making tortillas by hand. The mestiza's smiling image beckons from state-sponsored tourism advertisements, official and unofficial representations of Yucatecan folklore, and monuments in her honor in busy avenues in the capital city of Merida. Flesh-and-blood mestizas inhabit the rural and urban landscapes of Yucatan, engaging in commerce, raising children, keeping the ways of the *uuchbéen maako'ob* (the ancient ones). While the term *mestizo* everywhere else in Latin America has come to signify the ideology of blending of race and culture as a result of the colonial encounter, in Yucatan the word in its feminine form has become synonymous with "indigenous," "traditional," and—significantly for this book—"Maya."

Mestiza, an existing identity category, has been appropriated by the Yucatecan state in its promotion of indigenous culture by converting it into a "multicultural adornment," similar to what Andean indigenous anthropologist Silvia Rivera Cusicanqui (2012) describes in Bolivia. "Coloniality," a concept that accounts for racism as the organizing principle of the political economy of former colonies (Quijano 1992, 2000), is the continuation of colonial relationships in the absence of colonial structure. In its original elaboration, coloniality referred to the way in which race and capital intersect. As the concept has come to be further developed by Ramón Grosfoguel (2011a, 2011b) the colonial matrix of power, also referred to as the coloniality of power, describes the way in which coloniality is produced and reproduced through a matrix of social phenomena: gender, sexuality, religion, epistemology, authority, and legal institutions, among others. In this chapter, I consider how the coloniality of power manifests itself in local understandings of indigenous identity, poverty, and the Maya construct as they pertain to madness. These understandings, in turn, produce the social context of Las Lomas and its patients. Who is a Maya person in Yucatan? As I demonstrate in this chapter, this is an inherently colonial question. Nevertheless, local understandings of the indigenous people and culture of Yucatan must be addressed in a book about madness, coloniality, and modernity in the region. While this book is not a study of the Maya identity of Yucatan, the politics of heritage that have so powerfully caught the attention of scholars (Breglia 2006; Castañeda 1996; Armstrong-Fumero 2009, 2013; Barenboim 2018)[1] play a role in shaping the discourses of mental health and mental illness that circulate around Las Lomas. In this chapter, I lay the theoretical foundation guiding the rest of this book.

DECOLONIZING MAYA IDENTITY

During my first field visit to Yucatan in 2003, I lived in a small community of less than 300 people, which I call Yaxche', in the former henequen-producing (*agave fourcroydes*) region of Yucatan. Mamá Concha turned ninety-four that summer, and her family—six adult children who were now grandparents and even great-grandparents themselves—decided to throw her a party. Because I was staying at the home of one of her grandchildren, Candelaria, I was also invited. Mamá Concha's children went to great lengths to create a beautiful celebration for their mother: they killed several large hogs for *cochinita*, arranged for a priest to travel to the village to offer a mass in her honor, and banned all alcohol from the subsequent celebrations because she hated seeing her sons and grandsons get drunk. One last request was made of the women attending the party: everyone should wear her huipil.

Most young women in the family did not wear huipil every day, but everyone owned at least one. Most Yucatecan women, even white, elite women, own a huipil, a custom dating back at least 300 years. It is seen as entirely normal and appropriate to wear huipil in a variety of social settings and is not, on its own, seen as an indigenous identity marker. In Yaxche', women usually wore the huipil for the procession during the village *fiesta* in honor of the *Virgen de la Candelaria*, a major annual event. Luckily, I had brought my huipil with me to Yucatan, though I was missing a *pik*.[2] Candelaria took one of her late mother's old piks, added a few inches of fabric to the top, and I wore that. It was, however, a rare occasion for all the women in the family to wear huipil on the same day. Candelaria grumbled when she put her huipil on and discovered it was tighter than she wanted it to be; she had avoided wearing huipil for many years and had gained a little weight.

"Why don't you ever wear huipil?" I asked her as she pulled it off and started working on the dress's arm openings with a pair of scissors.

"I don't like it. The cut is too square, not flattering at all," she answered, needle and thread in her mouth, "I was a mestiza when I was a little girl, you know. But I became a *catrina* [a native Yucatec-Maya-speaking woman who was raised as a mestiza and decides to wear Western clothing instead of the huipil] when I went to the city to work."

Candelaria's nieces—Pamela, Olivia, and Daniela—all wore their *mini-huipil*, an updated version of the huipil popular among young women and shorter and narrower than the traditional one worn in this part of Yucatan. Olivia was very good at needlepoint sewing in *xook bi chuy*, a cross-stitch needlework style highly valued in Yucatecan textiles, and Pamela and Daniela looked admiringly at her recently completed huipil, a dainty and highly detailed splash of yellow and pink roses along the hem and collar, which was not too wide so as not to overwhelm the small dress. As I put on my own huipil, Carmen, Candelaria's sister-in-law, the girls' mother, clucked in approval and helped me pull it over the altered pik. Carmen is the only family member who wears huipil every day and self-identifies as a mestiza. Her son, Ramiro, came into the house as we were finishing up and exclaimed, "Beatriz, all you need is your *rebozo* [shawl] and you're all set! You'll be a real mestiza."

Momentarily confused, I turned to Carmen. "Should I wear a rebozo? I don't own one."

"Absolutely not!" she exclaimed, shooting a Ramiro an annoyed look, "rebozos are for the true mestizas [*las verdaderas mestizas*], not for you."

As soon as Carmen said this I realized what she meant. Yes, huipiles are worn by all kinds of women in a variety of social situations, but the only ones I have ever seen using a rebozo—outside of performances of the traditional *jarana* dance—are women who wear the huipil every day, women for whom wearing an huipil is not a day-to-day choice between an huipil and another kind of dress. Only mestizas wear huipil every day, and they nearly always accompany it with a rebozo. While it was socially acceptable for me to wear a huipil to Mamá Concha's party alongside the other women, wearing a rebozo would have violated local practice and been an unacceptable appropriation. I would have crossed the boundary from dressing to costuming.

As this vignette shows, the politics of *mestizaje* and indigenous identity in Yucatan are complicated, none more so than the mestiza identity category. The racial identity politics of Yucatan are unlike those of the United States, where race is traditionally understood as biological in foundation—evidenced by American hypodescent (the automatic assignment of children born from mixed-white and nonwhite unions to the nonwhite group) in defining legal blackness and U.S.

government concerns over blood quantum in defining Native American tribal affiliation for legal purposes. First, although the term mestizaje usually describes an ideology of identity that is neither indigenous nor European but conceived as a mixture of the two, in the Yucatecan context the word "mestiza" describes a very specific type of indigenous (Maya) identity. Mestizas, though frequently evoked as the symbol of Maya indigeneity, are not the only indigenous women in Yucatan. A mestiza identifies herself primarily by the clothing she wears and her fluency in Yucatec Mayan. She can stop being a mestiza—and become a catrina— by simply choosing to no longer wear the huipil. But while there seems to be some flexibility in the ability of a mestiza to stop being a mestiza, this flexibility does not work the other way around, particularly for non-Yucatec-speaking women—although a catrina may go back to being a mestiza, a girl who has never been a mestiza cannot become one simply by wearing the huipil. Moreover, while all mestizas are indigenous, not all indigenous women are mestizas. Importantly, not all women who the anthropological gaze would recognize as indigenous would consider themselves as such.

The word "Maya" in Yaxche describes the language spoken by many but not all the people who live there. It is not a category of identity, though *Mayero* is used to describe people who speak Maya. Anthropologists and other scholars use the term Maya to describe indigenous peoples who speak or whose ancestors spoke one of twenty-nine related Maya languages, but the category itself loses meaning on the ground. While more robust in terms of its legal application, the term *indígena* (indigenous) is similarly complicated. There is no accepted absolute metric for who "counts" as indigenous in Mexico. A frequent metric has been whether a person is a speaker of Yucatec Mayan or another indigenous language. But many parents, in increasing numbers despite language revitalization efforts, are choosing not to teach their children the language. Another metric has been whether a person has a Maya surname or a Maya-speaking parent or grandparent. Yet many people in Yucatan who have Maya surnames or Maya-speaking parents or grandparents do not identify themselves as indigenous. Locally, as Armstrong-Fumero (2013) has pointed out, *de pueblo* (from a small town/village) is a much more relevant form of identification. The Maya identity of Yucatan is so contradictory and complex that several scholars, including me, have devoted pages to understanding it (Reyes-Foster 2012; Castañeda 2004; Hervik 2003; Castillo Cocom 2005).

The intersection of gender and indigeneity bears some discussion. Mestizas, the most visible representatives of Yucatec Maya indigeneity, typify other observations regarding the femininity of indigenous-gendered identity in Latin America (Martínez Novo 2003). Like other indigenous women, mestizas are fetishized in local and global imagination. As the chapter-opening lyrics of the song "La Mestiza" and various visual presentations suggest, the archetype of the mestiza is sensual, seductive, pure, friendly, nurturing, and mysterious. Likewise, local discursive representations of Maya men as drunkards (Reyes-Foster 2013b) parallel similar representations of indigenous men elsewhere (Gone 2014). As I discuss later in this chapter, in the Yucatan, an additional discursive representation exists that marks Maya men as suicidal. Yet even here, the femininity of indigenous suicide appears through the trope of Ixtab, the suicide goddess.

Local understandings of indigenous, Maya, and mestizo have a clear origin in Mexican revolutionary rhetoric and nation-building strategies. The agrarian revolution in Mexico was accompanied by Manuel Gamio's (2010) *indigenismo*, a strategy that aimed to hinge Mexican national identity on the Mexican people's indigenous heritage. However, this heritage was understood as a sort of obstacle to modernization—indigenismo was an assimilationist strategy that viewed mestizaje, an ideology of miscegenation, as the ideal Mexican "cosmic race" (Vasconcelos [1979] 1997). At the same time that indigenismo emerged as a driving ideology of national identity, Cárdenas's land reform transformed conditions on the ground for the inhabitants of Yaxche' and others like them, who continue to share the collective memory of esclavitud, albeit in often unintended ways (Fallaw 2001).

For many people in Yucatan, ethnicity is not an important category of identity. As Yucatec Maya anthropologist Juan Castillo Cocom notes, most rural Maya are more likely to identify themselves as supporters of one of the national political parties (PRI-ista, a follower of the PRI political party, or PAN-ista, a follower of the PAN political party), or by their communities of origin before they would identify themselves as indigenous or Maya. By the same token, *indio* remains a powerful racial epithet. Maya people face systematic exclusion and racism. Many are choosing to abandon their language and way of life in an effort to give their children better opportunities. For those children, many of them now grown, these opportunities have been elusive.

It may be apparent that while identity and understanding one's place in the world are important parts of daily life for many people in Yucatan, the identity categories social scientists rely on—Maya or indigenous—to label this population are seldom present on the ground and are insufficient to the task of understanding the way in which identity emerges as part of the colonial matrix of power. In fact, Juan Castillo Cocom (2005) has long argued that "Maya" as an ethnic category is a colonialist, oppressive construction. As he and others (Castañeda 2004; Reyes-Foster 2012; Watanabe and Fischer 2004) have observed, indigenous people who fall into the "Maya" category frequently do not self-identify as such but are more likely to identify with their communities of origin, language group, or political affiliation. The late twentieth century saw the emergence of the Pan-Maya movement in post–civil war Guatemala (Warren 1998), and in the twenty-first century, an organic Mayanist movement led by young people and greatly facilitated by social media has emerged in Yucatan as well, notably in resistance to state narratives of Maya identity and culture. A group of women Maya poets and writers maintains a vibrant writing collective. This movement, alongside other, smaller groups of people engaging in Maya identity work, suggests that local beliefs about Maya as ethnic and identity category are beginning to change.

One day in 2008, I was observing a group therapy session at Las Lomas. This particular session was for men and women who had been committed to Las Lomas following a suicide attempt. During this time, I came to know a young woman I refer to as Claudina. During a particularly emotional session, Claudina made a comment that crystalized my understanding of indigenous identity in Yucatan. Claudina shared the story of a recent breakup with a young man, who had left her for a woman who was a doctor. A hairstylist by trade, Claudina described her pain at comparing herself with the other woman, who she described as "elegant," presumably in contrast to herself. However, as she finished her story, she observed: "There is an elegance that comes from being a professional, and another that comes from mestizaje." Claudina spoke of her grandmother, a mestiza, as possessing a different kind of elegance from that of her rival.

When I analyzed Claudina's story (Reyes-Foster 2012), I saw her pain as a kind of grief work. Claudina knew she had neither the elegance of her rival nor that of her grandmother, whose status as a mestiza she deeply admired. She appeared to experience her own status—neither mestiza nor professional—as a loss, which crystalized intersections of gender, race, and class that clearly were important to identity work for non-Maya-speaking, non-huipil-wearing women like her. Put bluntly, Claudina was too *india*—a common epithet (with clear racial overtones) used in Mexico to label people as backward, ignorant, uncivilized—to be elegant like her rival, yet not Maya enough to be elegant like her mestiza grandmother.[3]

As a dark-skinned, non-Maya-speaking, urban-dwelling woman working a typical urban, working-class job, Claudina inhabits the gray space that frequently excludes people like her from the anthropological gaze on the Maya. Perhaps more importantly, that gray space excludes her for local representations and understandings of Maya people. If mestizas are the most visible representatives of Mayaness in Yucatan, people like Claudina are the most invisible. They face the same kind of systematic racism, exclusion, and discrimination that more visibly Maya people do, yet they are bereft of any of the advantages that accompany the cultural capital possessed by mestizas. In parallel, Claudina's experience is consistent with Silvia Rivera Cusicanqui's critique of Andean multiculturalism—when Maya identity is reduced to essentialist visions of rural life and huipil-clad mestizas, the ethnicity of Claudina and others like her is denied and erased (2010, 99).

Moreover, a powerful undercurrent in Claudina's story indexes the importance of social class in local identity. While Claudina describes her grandmother's elegance in terms of her ethnic identity, her rival's elegance is tied to her prestigious job as a doctor. Indeed, poverty is an important source of both identity and social belonging: rural Maya people frequently call themselves *le óotsil maako'ob* (the poor people) or *macehualo'ob* (the commoners).[4] While my interlocutors inside and outside Las Lomas spent very little time talking about their identities as indigenous or Maya people, their own poverty and that of others close to them was fuel for conversation.

Poverty is a powerful identity category because it reproduces social disparities in the most visible ways, particularly health disparities tied to poor governance. Back in Yaxche', in 2003—the same year Mamá Concha turned ninety-four—I met Chelito. A quiet young woman—she turned twenty-one that summer—with a quick smile, Chelito was thirty-five weeks pregnant when I met her, and I expected to congratulate her on the birth of her child before I left the field. A year prior, Chelito had suffered the second-trimester loss of her first child, and her husband and family eagerly, if anxiously, awaited the birth of her second. About a month after I met her, I left the village to visit family in Merida. When I came back, I ran into her sister, Ana, and asked after her.

"She has a bladder infection," Ana told me, "we took her to the clinic, but she should be coming home today. We thought she was in labor, but the doctors said she wasn't."

The next day, Carmen and I were chatting with Carmen's sister-in-law on the quiet road outside our house when something caught Carmen's attention. She looked down the road, to Chelito's house. The community ambulance had just pulled up outside. Carmen slowly shook her head.

"Something has happened," she said. We watched from afar as Chelito's mother and sister got out of the car. We could see they were holding a large flower arrangement. I heard the gravel crunching behind us, and I saw that another neighbor, Agustina, was walking our way.

"Días," she said in greeting.

A single, piercing shriek from down the road interrupted us before we could reply. "Oh, no," said Carmen, "That's Chelito's mother-in-law." The shriek turned into wailing.

Agustina nodded, her expression somber. "I'm going over there," she said, walking away from us, toward Chelito's house.

Carmen, her sister, and I looked at each other. The two quietly reminisced on the death of Chelito's first baby, and Carmen's sister recalled, in a very low voice, that just a few days before she went to the clinic, Chelito—a Jehovah's Witness - had been making fun of the saints on her mother-in-law's altar. We watched Agustina walk down the road, reach the home, and speak briefly with the people who had begun to gather there. A few minutes later, she walked back to us and confirmed our fears: Chelito's baby had died.

A few hours later, the ambulance returned, this time with Chelito's husband and a tiny white casket holding their infant son. As is customary, the home where Chelito and her husband resided with his mother and extended family was opened for the wake, and Carmen, her daughters, and I went to pay our respects. The single-room structure was a traditional clay, wood, and mud home with a corrugated cardboard roof (much cheaper than the traditionally used *huano* thatching, but also much hotter), and it was full of angry, grieving people. The white casket sat, empty, on the family's altar. The infant boy was in Ana's arms, wearing a new white outfit, wrapped in a blue blanket.

"The baby was alive yesterday," Ana cried between sobs, rocking him gently, "we *heard* him. We *felt* him move! Her private doctor said everything was fine, but the baby needed to be born. Then they *kept her*, at that clinic, for twelve hours! They said she was in labor. Then they said she wasn't. Then they said the baby was malnourished but *look at him*! This baby isn't malnourished. He's perfect."

She was right. The baby did not look premature or malnourished. He looked healthy. The pallor had not yet come to his face. Had he not been brought in a casket, we would have thought he was merely sleeping in his aunt's arms.

Ana tenderly ran her finger along his tiny eyebrows and nose. A male relative had found a video camera and was filming—Chelito was still recovering, she would not be back in time for her son's funeral, and she had been unconscious during surgery. She never had the opportunity to see or hold her son. She requested the wake and funeral be filmed so she could see it. Ana's chest heaved with a stifled sob. "Those doctors are *murderers*!" she cried in rage.

It was hard to understand what had happened. Chelito's family had made a significant financial sacrifice and hired a private obstetrician to monitor her pregnancy, though the birth would have to take place at el Seguro (IMSS), Mexico's socialized medical system for private employees.[5] Each month, she had visited IMSS for her prenatal appointment and saw her private obstetrician. Chelito had gone to her regular prenatal appointment with her private doctor, and the obstetrician had told them that although everything was fine, but if the baby was not born in the next week, they should go to the hospital. A few days later, she began to experience pain and, thinking she was in labor, she went to the medical center she was assigned to by IMSS just outside of Merida. Had her labor progressed normally, she would have had her baby there, but the medical center was not equipped to perform surgeries. Something happened in the twelve hours she was at the center, and her family never felt it got a straight answer. She developed a fever, and the staff told her she had a bladder infection, and the pain she was experiencing was not labor after all. Her family observed medical providers inject her pregnant belly, but no one ever explained what they were doing. During this time, the staff told Chelito and her family that the baby was probably malnourished and that her dates must be wrong, for the child was not full term yet. Twelve hours after she initially arrived, a panicked staff told them she needed to be transferred to the hospital in Merida for an emergency C-section in order to save the baby's life. By the time they got there, the baby had died.

Ana later told me the obstetrician who had performed the C-section was angry. The obstetrician told her that she suspected the baby was dead before Chelito had been sent to the hospital, that someone at the clinic had made a mistake, and the sudden rush had been to cover their tracks. She urged them to make a report to

Yucatan's human rights commission. This was the third stillborn baby that that particular clinic had sent her in a week. Contrary to the clinic staff's claim that the infant was malnourished or preterm, Chelito's baby son was a well-nourished, full-term infant. Her family ultimately did not pursue a human rights investigation, but they remain convinced that the infant was lost through medical neglect. Ana and Chelito immediately recognized that the clinic staff, seeing that they were poor, indigenous women from a remote village, had tried to convince them that they were somehow to blame by saying the baby was malnourished.

The day Chelito's baby died, Agustina, our neighbor, walked home with us from the wake. Her anger was palpable. "You see, Beatriz?" she said to me as we stopped at our home, "you see? Do you know why this happened?"

I shook my head.

"Because we're *poor*. Because that is all we can afford. Do you think Chelito's baby would have died if she could pay for a private hospital?"

Again, I shook my head. "No, I don't," I replied honestly.

"But the seguro? Bah! *Seguro que te mueres*! They think because we are poor our lives don't have any value. They just do what they want, without any account-ability. Nothing ever changes."

In 2003, Seguro Popular, Mexico's free or very cheap insurance option for those ineligible for IMSS, was on the cusp of coming into existence, but did not yet exist. Chelito was in fact quite fortunate that her husband had an employer willing to put him on his employment roll and pay for his access to IMSS. It was unusual for anyone in Yaxche' to have enough money to pay for a private physician. Despite their poverty, Chelito and her family had done everything they could to ensure a healthy pregnancy and birth, and yet not only were they denied this, they were blamed for the catastrophic outcome by the very medical institution that failed them. Agustina's words have stuck with me through the years because they revealed a painful awareness of the place of the poor in Mexican society: *because we are poor our lives don't have any value*. While Chelito's story took place outside of the context of mental health care, it perfectly illustrates the systemic problems in Mexican health care, problems that reproduce disparity and are observable across delivery of services, including in mental health care.

This keen understanding of the powerlessness poverty bestows is not unique to Yucatan. Poor people in many places understand the ways in which the struc-tural violence of capitalism acts upon their bodies (Scheper-Hughes 1985; Farmer 2004). Yet, while poverty presents a clearer and more identifiable identity cat-egory than *indígena* or Maya, the intersection between poverty and race is undeniable: people who are poor are also predominantly people considered indigenous in societal structure. Claudina understood this when she described the grief involved in inhabiting her identity category. Poverty was also a frequent subject of conversation and concern among my interlocutors inside the wards of Las Lomas.

Back at Las Lomas, in 2012, I met Brandon, a Maya-speaking young man who had attempted to commit suicide by hanging. Brandon was diagnosed with paranoid schizophrenia. His attending psychiatrist, Dr. Pacheco, asked him about what led him to his suicide attempt. Brandon talked about feeling "pressured," and the following conversation followed.

DR. PACHECO: Have you felt pressured in the past?
BRANDON: Well, once, in elementary school, the teacher assigned a paper that had to be typewritten. I will never forget my friend Ender who let me borrow his typewriter, because my dad didn't have money to pay for one [Brandon begins to weep]. That guy, he was my friend. I will never forget that.

[Dr. Pacheco reads over Brandon's file.]

DR. PACHECO: Why did you want to kill yourself, Brandon? Do you remember? Do you still want to die?
BRANDON: No, no.
DR. PACHECO: You do know you tried to kill yourself?
BRANDON: Yes, I tried to hang myself. But that isn't the way out.
DR. PACHECO: What is the way out?
BRANDON: To face my problems.
DR. PACHECO: Your family says you were closing all the windows in your home, saying the police were after you. Why was that?
BRANDON: Because of my own illness.
DR. PACHECO: Do you remember this happening, or do you not remember?
BRANDON: I don't remember.
DR. PACHECO: How are you feeling?
BRANDON: A little sad. I am remembering my childhood, the poverty.
DR. PACHECO: Does poverty make you sad?
BRANDON: Yes.

Poverty emerges as a source of pain for Brandon. While Dr. Pacheco had been focused on understanding the circumstances that led to Brandon's suicide attempt, and trying to gauge Brandon's presence of mind, Brandon's thoughts were focused on childhood memories of poverty.

As discussed in chapter 1, poverty is prevalent in Yucatan. Nearly 50 percent of the population lives in poverty; 10 percent lives in extreme poverty, according to CONEVAL, Mexico's social development agency (CONEVAL 2014). While there is evidence of a relationship between mental illness and poverty, the nature of this relationship is contested (Das et al. 2007; Lund et al. 2011). In their study of the relationship between poverty and mental illness across five countries, Das and colleagues found that in Mexico, mental health outcomes were actually *better* for the poor, not worse (Das et al. 2007, 475). This suggests that while poverty presents as a preoccupation in my ethnographic data, there is more to the story of mental illness and poverty in Mexico. This may be because although poverty is an important category of identity, familial unity plays an important role in treating mental illness. Most people who struggle with mental illness do not ever arrive at Las Lomas, and as I discussed in chapter 1, for those who do, family continues to play a key role. Brandon's mother, for instance, visited daily and told him that she was sleeping outside the hospital doors every night, so that he would feel that she was always with him. This was a lie that Dr. Pacheco disapproved of, but it made the hospital stay bearable for Brandon.

The previous discussion of the complexities of Maya identity illustrates some of the limits of current notions of coloniality, particularly as it pertains to indigeneity. Within the scholarship of coloniality, several dissenting voices may enable the construction of a conceptual framework to guide this book. As I described in chapter 1, Walter Mignolo argues that coloniality is part of what he terms "Western Modernity." However, Ramón Grosfoguel and Silvia Rivera Cusicanqui have taken Mignolo to task; Grosfoguel (2011a) argues that Mignolo and Quijano's coloniality is a universalizing concept and as such presents a colonizing discourse. Grosfoguel instead argues for epistemic plurality and the possibility of different ways of explaining and understanding the coloniality of power. On a related point, Rivera Cusicanqui accuses Mignolo of creating a self-contained circuit of power and knowledge that ignores and disempowers the contributions of scholars from the Global South:

> Yet, without altering anything of the relations of force in the "palaces" of the empire, the cultural studies departments in North American universities have adopted the ideas of subaltern studies and launched debates in Latin America, thus creating a jargon, a conceptual apparatus, and forms of reference and counterreference that have isolated academic treatises from any obligation or dialogue with insurgent social forces. Walter Mignolo and company have built a small empire within an empire, strategically appropriating the contributions of the subaltern studies school of India and the various Latin American variants of critical reflection on colonization and decolonization. (2012, 98)

Within this multivocal conversation exploring the coloniality of power/knowledge and how to best understand these competing discourses in the context of contemporary Yucatan, mestizaje presents a particular epistemic challenge, a challenge present in the literature.

On mestizaje, Chicana[6] feminist scholar Gloria Anzaldúa is perhaps best known for her book *Borderlands/La Frontera: The New Mestiza* (1987). In *Borderlands*, Anzaldúa introduces the logic of mestizaje alongside the concept of borderlands. Borderlands and border thinking present a possibility for thinking about boundaries and limits in identity categories in an open-ended manner, cognizant of the ways categories often thought of as discrete—indigenous and European—do not exist so separately in practice. Because of this, Mignolo and his followers (2000, 2003) have embraced Anzaldúa's vision of the mestiza as a decolonial option, a way to counter the epistemological erasure of indigenous thought by colonialism. Gabriela Ríos (2016) notes that Mignolo's embrace of borderlands has met resistance from North American indigenous scholars, who have critiqued mestizaje as a modern construct that is disengaged from indigenous epistemology or ontology, a critique that is voiced in similar ways by Rivera Cusicanqui (2010, 2012). However, although North American indigenous scholars reject Anzaldúa's mestizaje as product of modern logic, Rivera Cusicanqui (2010), in her view from the Global South, asserts that indigenous people have always had a claim to modernity. Reflecting on the history of indigenous rebellion, she notes "this demonstrates that we indigenous people were and are, above all, contemporary beings and peers, and in this dimension—*aka pacha*[7]—we realize and carry out our own stake in modernity" (5).

So while Mignolo's universalist argument sees alternative modernities as no less grounded in coloniality, Rivera Cusicanqui and others like Grosfoguel and de Sousa Santos argue for the possibilities of epistemic plurality that include indigenous and other modernities founded on epistemologies originating outside the Global North. If Quijano's original understanding of coloniality refers to the intersection of race and capital, Grosfoguel—building on the work of Fanon and Boaventura de Sousa Santos—proposes that in colonial societies, racialization occurs at the level of the body. A boundary separates what Fanon refers to as the zone of being—the zone inhabited by those whose race affords them power and privilege—and the zone of nonbeing (Fanon [1952] 2008). Grosfoguel then brings Fanon's zones of being and nonbeing into conversation with the work of Boaventura de Sousa Santos (2010). Grosfoguel argues that de Sousa Santos's description of the boundary between rich and poor in modernity as an "abysmal line" should be understood as the demarcation of the zones of being and nonbeing (2011b, 100). To follow his thinking, the line between the colonizer and the colonized is insurmountable, although varying degrees of intersectional privilege occur within each zone.

Grosfoguel's concept is useful for understanding colonialism and modernity—these zones are relationships, not geographical locations, thus the concept can be used to analyze Pedro González Casanova's (1969) original idea of "internal colonialism." However, Yucatan presents a real challenge because of the blurring of its identity boundaries, as the previous excerpts show. The complexity of indigenous identity in Yucatan makes it difficult to answer the question frequently asked when I discuss my research with others: How many of your informants were Maya? Sometimes, the answer seems to be "none of them." Other times, the answer seems to be "all of them." One can argue that Yucatan is full of Mayas who are not indigenous (Castañeda 2004) and Mayas who are not Mayas (Castillo Cocom 2005), and non-Mayas who claim Maya identity, and Mayas who are fighting to be called Maya. Although the focus of this book is not identity, the subject keeps appearing when trying to make sense of the narrative of Yucatan's Maya heritage and how it relates to the pressing question of mental health.

A clear understanding of the relationship between identity, coloniality, and madness is necessary to understand the subject at hand. While Fanon's use of zones of being and nonbeing was limited to defining the line between colonizer and colonized, I argue that sanity and madness can also be understood using this framework. The sane are in the zone of being. Those deemed "mad" are zoned into nonbeing: they are uniquely vulnerable, as they lose all rights to self-determination when they are confined. The previous ethnographic examples demonstrate that while colonial logics are constantly at play inside and outside the psychiatric ward, the irreconcilable abyss between colonizer and colonized described by Grosfoguel falls short as an explanatory framework. I propose another way to see this framework. Unlike French and English, Spanish recognizes two different modalities of being: *ser*, which is permanent, and *estar*, which is temporary. I suggest that in Yucatan, alongside *la zona del ser y la zona del no-ser, también tenemos la Zona del Estar* (alongside the zone of being and the zone of nonbeing, we also have the zone of "estar" [conditional form of the verb "to be"]).[8]

La Zona del Estar exists as an area of flux and change within the colonial matrix of power. The concept is characterized by a temporality of constant present, allowing for the coexistence of multiple ways of being-in-the world. Three scholars of coloniality have proposed similar notions of understanding time. The first, Boaventura de Sousa Santos (2010), proposes a "sociology of absence" founded on an expansion of the present to allow for the emergence of epistemic pluralities. The second, Silvia Rivera Cusicanqui (2010), writes of *aka pacha*, an indigenous temporality characterized by a constant, cyclical present. The third concept was proposed by Juan Castillo Cocom and colleagues in response to notions of Maya ethnogenesis in Yucatan. The concept of ethnoexodus (Castillo Cocom, Rodriguez, and Ashenbrender 2017) rejects the notion that identities have points of origin and bounded existences, positing that identities are entered and exited at will at different points in time in different ways.

Ethnoexodus, aka pacha and the sociology of absence all present useful decolonial ways of thinking about time. One way in which the Zona del Estar is different is that it is not all-encompassing: subjects can enter and exit this zone, though not always at will. La Zona del Estar bridges the abyss between the zona del ser and zona del no-ser. It explains the shifting nature of indigenous identity without minimizing the reality of colonial violence or erasing indigenous bodies and culture. It is an anti-essentialist, anti-homogenizing theoretical tool that lends itself particularly well for thinking through indigenous identity and madness in Yucatan.

Madness and indigeneity, both products of the colonial matrix of power, exist in the Zona del Estar.

The temporality of the Zona del Estar allows for the shifting and overlap of identity performances while at the same time as it attends to the fact that this temporality is always mediated by the coloniality of power. When Maya people are those who speak Maya or dress a certain way, they are fetishized: their textiles, language, and images are commodified for tourist consumption with little attention to the everyday racism and discrimination to which they are subjected. When Maya people are those whose parents speak Maya or dress a certain way, but who choose to speak Spanish, abandon traditional dress, and raise their children to speak Spanish, they may be doing so because they believe disavowing these "markers" of Maya-ness will allow them to overcome the racism, discrimination, and poverty experienced by their parents. Yet they soon find that they experience racism, discrimination, and poverty nonetheless. When people like Claudina grow up with Maya-speaking grandmothers and parents who reject Maya language and culture, they often experience a profound sense of loss, an ambivalent grief of something missing and replaced with something worse: losing the mestiza, but not the *India*. This all occurs in the Zona del Estar, as identity shifts and wanes through internal and external forces. The concept is also useful for thinking about everyday existence in the psychiatric hospital. The line between sanity and madness is also colonial.

In much the same way that colonizer and colonized are zoned into being and nonbeing, a similar line exists between the sane and the mad. The mad are routinely zoned into nonbeing: their rights are stripped, their voices ignored, their bodies violated and disciplined. Las Lomas is the Zona del Estar between sanity and madness: linear time loses meaning, giving way to a permanent sense of present. In my previous work (Reyes-Foster 2016b), which I will revisit in chapter 6, I have written about how people in the acute ward exist in registers of visibility, making themselves visible and invisible to their medical providers. This notion of a register of visibility is possible because of the temporality of the psychiatric ward. When patients enter Las Lomas—particularly when they find themselves in the acute ward—they enter a zone characterized by a constant present: decisions made on a day-to-day basis, without thoughts about the future.[9] Symptoms are assessed, medications are adjusted, and when the patients' condition begins to change—that is, when they no longer fall into the parameters of madness—attending physicians begin to contemplate the future and the possibility of releasing them. In this sense, the patients begin to exit the Zona del Estar of madness.

La Zona del Estar bears some similarities to Castillo Cocom and colleagues' notion of ethnoexodus. Ethnoexodus contains an inherent possibility of entrance and exit: subjects go "in and out" of particular identities, folding and unfolding in response to particular circumstances. Both concepts present a way for thinking through transitory "in-betweenness," although they are arrived at in different ways, the first in response to scholarship of ethnogenesis, the second building more directly on scholarship of coloniality. Ethnoexodus is critical of the notion of *ethnos* as belonging and the idea that ethnic identities are stable or have identifiable points of emergence (genesis). This concept is quite useful when thinking about Maya identity in Yucatan. In a complementary way, La Zona del Estar focuses on the role of temporality within these shifts in identity while remaining attentive to the power dynamics inherent in the colonial matrix of power. Because of its engagement with temporality, the concept also readily lends itself to analyzing mental illness and mental institutions.[10]

MAYA APOCALYPSE AND ETHNOGRAPHIC ENTRAPMENT EN LA ZONA DEL ESTAR

Maya culture holds great monetary value to the Yucatecan state, which has, since the turn of the century, embraced tourism as an economic development strategy. These activities seemed to come to a frenzy as things moved closer and closer to December 21, 2012, the date of the alleged Maya apocalypse. The "Mayan Apocalypse" was a discursive motif that emerged at the turn of the twenty-first century, initially among practitioners of New Age religions and then spreading as the date drew nearer.

The idea that the Maya calendar had an end date of December 21, 2012 (solstice) is based on a misunderstanding of Maya calendrics. The ancient Maya had a complex calendar that included several different ways of accounting for time. One of these, the Long Count calendar, is comprised of a grand cycle of thirteen Bak'tuns (one Bak'tun being a period of 144,000) or about 5,125 years (Carlson 2011). It was this cycle that came to an end in 2012. Although archaeologists (Restall and Solari 2011; Carlson 2011) noted that Maya time, being cyclical, would simply begin a new Bak'tun at the end of an old one, the "end of the Maya calendar" inspired a slew of apocalyptic commentary in the Global North.

In the United States, the History Channel started airing "2012 prophesy" programming as early as 2009, linking the Maya calendar to figures like Nostradamus and the book of Revelations. A blockbuster film about a worldwide environmental catastrophe titled *2012* (Emmerich 2009), bearing no connection to Maya people or culture, was released. With the emergence of social media, cultural commentary about the alleged Maya apocalypse went viral, prompting serious institutions like NASA to put out a press releases addressing it (NASA 2012) and news organizations like National Public Radio to cover it. Skeptics joyfully made fun of believers, and archaeologists such as Arlen Chase, William Saturno, and Lisa Lucero (Roach 2011; Vergano 2012) attempted to shift the narrative away from misinterpretations of ancient Maya culture toward a greater appreciation of the civilization in general. In one 2012-themed program, archaeologist Arlen Chase appeared in an interview and stated matter-of-factly, "What's going to happen on December 21, 2012? Uhh, nothing!"

Eschatological fantasy is an important motif in Abrahamic traditions, especially Christianity, and this fantasy has frequently bled into U.S. and Mexican popular culture: end-times concerns emerged near July 1997 in connection to Nostradamus, again at the turn of the millennium, and then again around the date of June 6, 2006. Meanwhile, followers of New Age religions have long obsessed over the Maya calendar and its connection to the dawning of the New Age (Castañeda 1996). The Maya were already associated with certain mystery: despite attempts by many people, including Maya people themselves, to counter it, the popular misconception that Maya civilization suddenly vanished, and Maya people mysteriously disappeared, remains a stubborn urban tale. Compounded with preexisting notions of this mysterious collapse (Stromberg 2012), the Maya Apocalypse encouraged newfound interest in the so-called Maya region, of which Yucatan was home of several UNESCO World Heritage Sites such as the ruins of Chichén Itzá and Uxmal, and the state was ready to seize this opportunity to encourage an increase in tourism revenues. Anticipated increases in tourism revenues resulted in the building of an expansive, world-class museum so expensive it is virtually inaccessible to the local population outside of the middle and upper classes. In addition, the Yucatecan state sponsored and organized an "International Festival of Maya Culture," although it featured no Maya people. Millions of dollars were spent renovating the welcome centers at the most well-known archaeological sites that were expected to draw the largest numbers of tourists. The site of Chichén Itzá inaugurated a state-of-the art "Light and Sound" show, and the artist Yanni gave a concert in the "magical city" of Izamal.

Alongside these developments, in the first decade of the twenty-first century, the Yucatecan state opened a new university, Universidad de Oriente, in the city of Valladolid. The university embraced an intercultural model of education, featuring bilingual signage in Spanish and Yucatec Mayan. Its target population was first-generation Maya students from the eastern side of the peninsula. Universidad de Oriente's three inaugural majors were closely tied to the state's strategic interest in economic development through tourism: culinary arts, tourism, and Maya language and culture.

In response to newfound state investment in Maya culture and the state-sponsored International Festival of Maya Culture in particular, in 2012 a group of self-identified Maya created a counter-festival that they called the "Independent Festival of Maya Culture," which featured music, poetry readings, and academic panels hosted in small towns throughout the state. The festival resulted in the creation of Colectivo Cha'anil Kaaj, "an open, diverse and heterogenous group with clear objectives: to make the contemporary Maya people visible, have its voice heard through its own means, and recover spaces that have been violently taken"

(Cha'anil Kaaj 2015). Maya activists invested in identity politics see this embrace of Maya identity as inherently decolonial.

Renewed attention to Maya culture and Maya heritage has added a layer of complexity and bigger stakes for both the local population and the state. In the twenty-first century, the preservation and revitalization of Yucatec Maya language and culture have become urgent as Maya linguists warn that the language is becoming endangered. This urgency is predicated on a particular idea about what Maya culture is and what it should look like, an idea that appears to be based on a static understanding of culture in general and Maya-ness in particular. By the same token, the concern over the gradual endangerment of the Maya language also reflects a recognition of the racist colonialist structures that have created the conditions for the language to disappear. Nascent identity movements embraced by many young people, such as Cha'anil Kaaj and the emergence of an artistic renaissance among Maya youth (Martineau 2014; Villegas 2016), point to an encouraging shift in thinking about Maya language and indigenous identity. This broader social context shapes and is shaped by the ever-changing present of the Zona del Estar. When it comes to indigenous identity, the Zona del Estar is further entangled in the snare of ethnographic entrapment.

Ethnographic entrapment gained salience in North American Indian scholarship (Simpson 2014; Smith 2014; de Silva 2007), especially in its critique of anthropological complicity with settler colonialism.[11] In the logic of ethnographic entrapment, Native peoples are recognized as worthy only when they reify their otherness in accordance with a white gaze—in other words, only when they affirm fetishized notions of indigeneity such as speaking an indigenous language, wearing indigenous clothing, or engaging in "traditionally indigenous" activities. Ethnographic entrapment describes the conditions criticized by Rivera Cusicanqui when she notes that the ethnicity of indigenous people in South America is erased when they do not conform to a particular view of what "being indigenous" means.

Indigenous scholars have rightly noted the role of anthropologists in the creation of ethnographic entrapment, as acknowledged by native and nonnative anthropologists themselves (Arndt 2016; Briggs and Bauman 1999; Simpson 2007, 2014). Audra Simpson argues that the ethnographic gaze results in a "narrow, ritualistic, and procedural" (2007, 98) representation of indigenous people that frequently bears little resemblance to what is witnessed by ethnographers on the ground yet holds an authenticating power. This power results in the devaluing of difference as "confusion" or "forgetting" on the part of indigenous people. As a result, divergence from this original "authentic" representation of indigeneity is not recognizable to the anthropological gaze as indigenous. Ethnographic entrapment is thus the scholarly reification of one version of indigenous existence as real or authentic versus another. Simpson points out that "concepts have teeth, and teeth that bite through time" (100), and what exists in scholarly writing can have real-world consequences.

As evidenced by the works of Silvia Rivera Cusicanqui writing on South America and Castillo Cocom writing on Yucatan, this critique holds ground outside the North American Indian context. Castillo Cocom (2005) identifies the "Maya" as a conceptual category created by scholars in the Global North and (ab)used by the Mexican and Yucatecan state. Playing with the K'ichee' Maya creation story, the *Popol Vuh*, in which humans and the earth are portrayed as the fourth attempt at creation by the gods, Castillo Cocom posits that new "gods"— anthropologists, historians, linguists, and archaeologists—created the "Maya" as they are written about today: "[They] dialogue between themselves to figure out *what* Maya culture is, *who* is Maya and *why*. Yes, there was dialogue: but only after the gods created the Maya did they talk to the 'Maya' they created. And then the 'Maya' *talked back*" (132, emphasis in original). Castillo Cocom argues that the invented ethnic category of "Maya" is an oppressive, essentializing tool exploited by the state—much in the same sense that Simpson talks about the way in which anthropological writings on indigenous peoples were used to justify their dispossession.

Importantly, in Castillo Cocom's narrative, one can see experiences that can be arguably read as ethnographic entrapment and an effort to "talk back" to the creators of the Maya in a way that does not reify entrapment. He does this by writing in a style that is purposefully disjointed and, in his words, as "schizophrenic" as his own identity:

> I am bordering on schizophrenia. I "meet" myself in the midst of many I's that are watching me. They transform me one by one and all at once as if they were a strange chorus of the unknown and unwanted. . . . Sometimes I think I am talking to the gods, but my friends at 7-Eleven in the *plaza* of Mérida tell me they are only anthropologists. Sometimes I think I am talking to an anthropologist and it is just myself. . . . Sometimes I am a Maya and sometimes I am a post-Maya. I am also a Mayanist or *mayista* and at other times a post-Mayanist. . . . I am a sociologist, Indígena, anthropologist, Mexican, Yucateco and none of these things. "I" am vulnerable. I *observe* my Self as a "vulnerable observed." (2005: 132–133)

One could argue that Castillo Cocom's writing style is another way to engage in Simpson's call for *ethnographic refusal*, a conscious setting of limits by the anthropologist and the people she works with. For Simpson, this refusal takes the form of silence and things left unsaid. For Castillo Cocom, this refusal is an outright challenge disguised in playful writing, a deliberate strategy acknowledged in one of his own publications (Castillo Cocom, Rodriguez, and Ashenbrender 2017). This refusal has at times been more forthright. In a footnote in a different article, Castillo Cocom and Ríos Luviano (2012) speak to a request from someone who I assume is an anonymous reviewer, concerning a claim they make about the colonial nature of Indian performance: "Do we need a reference here? A citation? Or, is it you—is it you who needs a citation? Very well then, but which one should it be? . . . Which one confirms your belief in our analysis? Which one confirms our status in your imagined circuits of our power/knowledge?" (253).

In this coauthored article, Castillo Cocom and Ríos Luviano (2012) continue their crusade against the hypocrisies of state-sanctioned Maya-ness, turning their attention to "Maya Dignitaries"—"officials created by Mexican Law as a means to revitalize and support indigenous Maya Culture" (229)—in Quintana Roo, Yucatan's neighboring state. According to Castillo Cocom and Ríos Luviano, these legal positions were created to allow Maya people to resolve internal problems using a preexisting—pre-Colombian—legal system, yet it was unclear from where the Quintana Roo state legislature derived its assumptions about what this legal system should look like. In the end, Castillo Cocom and Ríos Luviano argue that the Maya Dignitaries are a ruse, "smoke and mirrors," and a "one-trick pony," meant to further the state's agenda by essentializing Maya culture (241). It is here that Castillo Cocom and Ríos Luviano identify the performative nature of the task: "Do they know that the state's portraiture of them as Maya, like Warhol's painting of Russell Means, 'is not an Indian'? Can they recognize that their performance of Indian is a colonial simulation?" (241).

Performance—and the performative nature of Maya identity—plays an important role in Castillo Cocom's writings. Like gender identity (Butler 1999 [1990]), ethnic identity is something one *does*, not something one *has*. Like gender identity, ethnic identity is simultaneously enacted and imposed. If, as Butler notes, the gendered body "has no ontological status apart from the various acts which constitute its reality" (1999 [1990], 185), the same holds true for the ethnicized body: its only reality is that of the actions that constitute it. My claim is that ethnographic entrapment is constituted through its performative demands on the indigenous subject: if Maya are only Maya when they fit into a particular aesthetic, the ability to perform Maya-ness is central to their own societal value as Maya. Worse still, if they are not valued as Mayas, they are devalued as *indios*. This is the perversity of ethnographic entrapment in Yucatan: perform the desired aesthetic of the Maya subject—wear the clothing, speak the language, do the ceremonies—or be an indio. Ethnographic entrapment occurs within the Zona del Estar; despite the fact that identities are ever-changing and flexible, they remain mediated by a hierarchically defined colonial matrix. The "bite" of the anthropological "Maya" is Claudina's ambivalent grief in the Zona del Estar: she does not have the flexibility to enter or exit Maya identity. This flexibility has been taken from her.

HERITAGE AND THE SUICIDAL MAYA

JANUARY 2008

It is a hot, muggy morning. At least, it feels hot and muggy to me, but considering I arrived just a few days ago from a frigid New Jersey winter, it is hard to tell. I know that in a week or two the heat and the mugginess will fade into the background and become invisible. My cousin invited me to accompany her to a cultural function at the Escuela de Artes de Yucatan (ESAY), her employer. A belly dancer from India is giving a presentation. ESAY is located in the building of the now-defunct Merida train station. Across the street, I spy a hotel that rents rooms by the hour. Facing the hotel, a fruit vendor is selling citrus fruits, oranges and grapefruits cut up, bagged up with jicama, a sweet root known as the Mexican potato, drizzled with lime juice and sprinkled with red chili powder. The building has been beautifully restored, the crown jewel of a flurry of spending on education that characterized the recently ousted PAN (Partido Acción Nacional) administration.

I have been in Yucatan for three days now. I am anxious to start my work. But today, I am enjoying the performance. The audience, my cousin tells me, is made up of students, ESAY employees, and their families. When the event ends, my cousin introduces me to a man whose name I forget almost immediately. This is the first and last time I will ever see him. My cousin explains to me that he is a sociologist at the local social science research center of the Universidad Nacional Autónoma de México (UNAM). He is a *waach*, a *chilango*, a man from México City. As a foreigner, he represents all that my Yucateco friends despise: the fast speech, the swagger, the gregarious attitude that in other parts of México and in the United States would be interpreted as friendliness but here is seen as arrogance and a false sense of entitlement. Yucatecos are quiet people. They don't like false friendliness. They don't appreciate people who make themselves comfortable before they are invited to do so. They especially don't like *waaches* from México City, who move to the quiet Yucatan and bring with them their crime, their unruliness, and their despicable driving habits.

He shakes my hand firmly and my cousin introduces me. "This is my cousin, Beatriz, she's doing her thesis research on suicide."

The man's eyes light up. "Really? That's a great topic! Did you know Yucatan occupies the first place nationally in suicides? They say it's something about the local Maya culture." (Field notes, January 2008)

This was probably the fifth time in three days that someone had shared this mistaken bit of data with me. What was remarkable at the time, and still remains so, was the fact that this belief—indigenous people in Yucatan are suicidal— seemed to be prevalent among city-dwellers in Merida; when I went to other parts of the state, suicide was not described as particularly prevalent nor part of local culture.

A caveat is warranted here. Yucatan's suicide rate is higher than the national average. When I conducted my field research in 2008, the suicide rate in Yucatan was 9.2 per 100,000 people, nearly double the national average of 4 per 100,000 people. Yucatan's suicide rate has always remained relatively stable and is comparable to that of the United States, which usually averages about 10 per 100,000.

This is *not* to say that suicide is not of concern in Yucatan, particularly as research has shown the crisis of suicide among indigenous peoples in the American continent (Stevenson 2014; Kral 2012). My research with surviving family members of people who committed suicide and with people who attempted suicide shows that suicide is a tragic event that brings unspeakable pain to those affected by it. But, just as in the United States, we do not ponder the cultural reasons for our suicide rate, and neither should we in Yucatan. People in Yucatan commit suicide for many reasons, and although "culture" may play a role, there is no "Maya mystery" to resolve. Suicide is generally linked to suffering.[12]

In the contested space where the politics of identity meet the politics of heritage, I found myself trying to study mental illness.[13] Anthropological approaches, which see heritage as a process, tend to focus on how the material culture of the past is used and evaluated in the present. The usefulness of heritage to furthering the agenda of the state is clear. Because heritage is tied up in the relationships between the people who interact with it—including those, like the mestiza, who are transformed into the very embodiment of heritage—it is an ambivalent and contested arena of interaction. This should be apparent in the state's wholehearted investment in the preservation of Maya culture and the ways in which various players have reacted to it.[14]

Perhaps at this point the reader is wondering how this discussion of heritage relates to mental health or psychiatry. It is here where Maya heritage, Maya identity, and my own research on suicide and mental health converge. My initial interest in suicide emerged precisely because of the belief, stated by many Yucatecans I encountered over my years of research in Yucatan, that Maya people were prone to suicide. When I began studying Maya culture more seriously, I was initially taken aback by Diego de Landa's 1566 description of a suicide goddess, Ixtab, who, he wrote, would take those who hanged themselves to a sort of heaven (Tozzer 1941). In another seventeenth-century text, *Informe Contra Idolorum Cultures*, Pedro Sánchez de Aguilar ([1639] 2003) describes the indigenous people of Yucatan as highly susceptible to suicide by hanging. When I traveled to Merida, I was greeted by imagery of the alleged deity, whom Landa calls Ixtab. Alfred Tozzer's 1941 annotated edition of Landa's *Relación de las Cosas de Yucatan* remains the most complete academic edition of this work. In a footnote to the passage where Landa describes Ixtab, Tozzer speculates that a particular iconographic figure found in one of the surviving Maya books, the Dresden Codex, is a likely representation of the deity. This image (Image 2) depicts a young woman hanging from a sky band by the neck, her eyes closed, and her body covered in death spots. I found the image featured in museums and tourist art, but also in local children's literature (Image 3) and other forms of media meant for local consumption (Reyes-Foster and Kangas 2016; Reyes-Foster 2013b). The name "Ixtab" also appeared in headlines of suicides splashed on the front pages of local *nota roja* newspapers (Reyes-Foster 2013b).[15] When I began dissertation fieldwork in

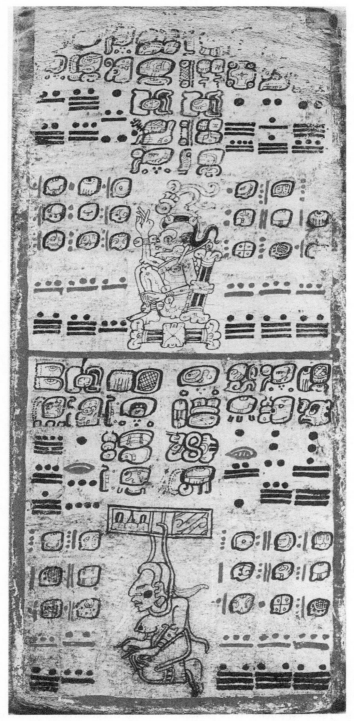

FIGURE 2. Iconographic depiction of moon goddess believed to be Ixtab from the Dresden Codex (53b). Courtesy of *Ancient Americas* at LACMA.

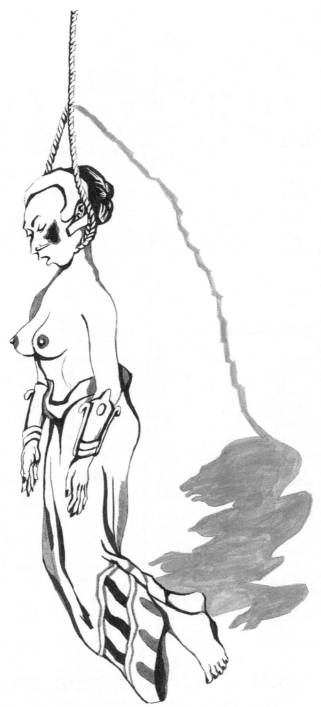

FIGURE 3. Stylized depiction of Ixtab published in a children's book. Artist: Juan Ramón Chan. Courtesy of Editorial Dante.

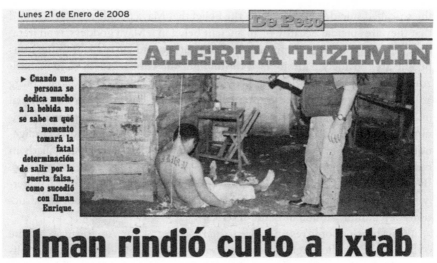

FIGURE 4. "Ilmán Rindió Culto a Ixtab," newspaper article in *De Peso*. January 2008.

January 2008, I was interested in suicide as a Maya problem, particularly whether suicide was somehow more acceptable in Yucatan because of its Maya heritage and identity. In this sense, I was misguided by my own expectations of Maya culture and experienced my own "settler agnosia" (Arndt 2016, 466).

Soon enough, however, I noticed that what circulated in local discourse was not quite reflected on the ground. As I state earlier in this section, suicide was not a "cultural" matter in Yucatan. The people I spoke with throughout the state, whether or not they had been personally impacted by suicide, did not view it as the product of cultural attitudes. Nobody spoke of a suicide goddess. Suicide remained a highly stigmatized form of death, viewed as neither acceptable nor understandable. One way in which local understandings of suicide were remarkable was that suicide was not viewed as the result of agency but more frequently of demonic intervention (Reyes-Foster 2013a), but this view was not part of local public discourses about suicide. Upon further research, I found little evidence of the existence of an actual Maya suicide deity—it is likely that Landa's interpretation of Ixtab was incorrect, as there is no evidence of prevalent hanging or of a hanging-associated goddess in Maya iconography, and archaeologists and iconographers agree that the woman hanging from the sky band in the Dresden Codex is more likely a manifestation of the moon goddess during a lunar eclipse (Reyes-Foster and Kangas 2016). It turned out that suicide could not be understood as a problem of "ancient Maya culture" after all.

The idea that Maya people are suicidal is most likely not an intentional part of the state's tourism development strategy. However, the frameworks I have outlined in this chapter make the discursive link between suicide, Maya people, and the so-called suicide goddess clear. The belief that Maya people are suicidal, and that they are suicidal because of an ancient belief in a Maya goddess, is an iteration of ethnographic entrapment. The ways of life and customs of indigenous people are routinely pathologized throughout the Global North (Greensmith 2012; Blagg 2016), with indigenous people frequently portrayed as alcoholic (Blagg 2016; Reyes-Foster 2013b) or emotionally unstable (Gone 2014). In the colonial imaginary of the Maya, we see the enduring representation of indigenous femininity in the figure of the mestiza contrasting with the representation of indigenous masculinity in the portrayal of the drunken, suicidal indio, particularly in red or tabloid journalism, as I discuss in my previous work (Reyes-Foster 2013b). By the same token, these discursive portrayals of indigenous people reveal underlying understandings of femininity that parallel but also differ from constructions of femininity found in Latin America.

While bearing some resemblance to *marianismo*, a Latin American archetype of Spanish Catholic origin that characterizes ideal femininity as chaste, self-sacrificing, and nurturing, the mestiza archetype is also characterized by sensuality and mystery. This is exemplified in the origin story of the Yucatecan demon, *La Xtabay*. In the story, two women of equal beauty, Xkeban and Utzcolel, live in a village and die on the same day. Xkeban is free with her physical affections and socially ostracized as a prostitute, yet a kind and caring human being. Utzcolel is a paragon of womanly virtue, yet cold and cruel in disposition. When the women die, Xkeban's corpse releases a sweet aroma, and from the soil of her grave sprouts the beautiful, fragrant flower, *Xtabentún* (*Turbina corymbosa*). In contrast, Utzcolel's corpse decomposes immediately, releasing a fetid, unbearable stench. From her grave, a thorny *Tzacam* (*Nopalea gaumeri*) cactus sprouted. Both Utzcolel and Xkeban are mestizas: the story's moral is that kindness and purity of spirit are more important than sexual virtue and a chaste reputation. The story contrasts with traditional Latin American marianismo, which draws sharp distinctions between *mujeres de la casa*, who are sexually inexperienced, and *mujeres de la calle*, who are promiscuous.

However, the story does not end there. Although there are competing versions, all agree that while Xkeban's legacy is the *Xtabentun* flower from which a liqueur of the same name is made, Utzcolel's angry spirit transformed into a demon known as Xtabay, who appears in the guise of a beautiful woman dressed in white and lures drunk men into an uncertain fate. In some versions of the story, a drunk man follows the beautiful woman, and when he finally reaches her and embraces her, he finds he is embracing the thorny *Tzacam*. In other versions, the man's fate is more sinister; he is strangled by the Xtabay, whose name translates to "the ensnarer."[16] The drunken Maya meets a female personification of death.

The entanglement of Maya heritage and Maya identity becomes evident here: "the Maya" may be "invented," as Castillo Cocom claims, yet the indigenous foundation of this invention was not conjured from nowhere, and neither was the mestiza. What is invented—better yet, forced together—is the linkage between ancient Maya material culture and contemporary organic expressions of identity. The connection between contemporary suicide and the misinterpreted Ixtab is a by-product of the Maya invention and Yucatan's heritage-as-practice. It is a form of ethnographic entrapment that takes the invention of Maya culture and uses it to pathologize indigenous identity and situate suicide as a cultural rather than structural problem.

DE REGRESO A LA ZONA DEL ESTAR

Fanon once said that colonization was a great purveyor to psychiatric hospitals (2004 [1961]). By this, he was referring to the psycho-affective effects of the colonial experience, which resulted in a variety of psychiatric symptoms, some of which he documented in the context of the Algerian War in *The Wretched of the Earth*. Fanon believed that colonization constituted the systematic negation of the humanity of the colonized. This negation reduced colonial life to mere existence: "to live simply means not to die" (2004, 232). It is the negation that is the foundation of the zones of being and nonbeing (Fanon 2008 [1952]), which in turn are interpreted by Grosfoguel (2011b) as being separated by an insurmountable abyss. Simultaneously, we can see the colonial matrix of power as defined by the intersections of race and capital, with its accompanying effects on labor, gender, sexuality, social class, and religion. The zones of being and nonbeing live inside the colonial matrix of power. Within this matrix, notions of rationality, self-sufficiency, and subjectivity arise, always mediated by whether they are experienced by subjects in either zone. The Zona del Estar emerges from the colonial matrix of power, superimposed like another layer of reality over the chasm separating the zones of being and nonbeing.

Madness presents an opportunity for fugue, an escape to a different temporality—yet people considered mad are remarkably vulnerable. At Las Lomas, those vulnerable people are subjected to involuntary treatment, physical restraining, and restriction on their movement as a matter of course. They are vulnerable to physical and sexual abuse from hospital employees and other patients—while there were no allegations of misconduct during my research at Las Lomas, I heard stories whispered behind closed doors of psychotic patients in the past who had been subjected to these abuses and were subsequently disbelieved by their doctors and family members. Dr. Tun told me of a woman who kept saying she was being raped by the devil each night. It was eventually discovered that one of the overnight staff members had been sexually assaulting her. Thus, while one might argue that the Zona del Estar accounts for gray areas between colonizer and colonized, it also remains firmly entrenched in the colonial matrix of power. It does not negate the zones of being and nonbeing; it merely explores a way in which the two are bridged.

The Zona del Estar can help make sense of the flexibility of indigenous identity while it accounts for the way this flexibility is limited. A young mestiza can choose to put up her huipil and wear Western clothing. She may even find comfort in fading into the background alongside the other young brown women riding the bus to Merida. Perhaps she hopes she will meet a good man with stable work, and together they will raise children who will not know hunger. Maybe she will try to teach her children Maya, but when they stubbornly speak back to her in Spanish, she will throw her hands in the air. After all, Spanish is the language they need to succeed. One day, her little boy will come home with tears in his eyes because his friend called him an indio, and she will wipe his tears away and tell him not to mind him and focus on his studies without revealing the hurt she feels for him. When her boy grows up, he will have little to connect him to his mother's culture. He will not speak Maya, although he might understand it, and he won't know the first thing about making *milpa*. He will love his mother but be embarrassed by the fact that she is *de pueblo*, a euphemism for indigenous (Armstrong-Fumero 2009). His own dark-skinned daughter will look wistfully at her light-skinned friends, who look like the people on TV, and she will wish she, too, had light hair and skin.

This is the context in which I began my ethnographic experience at Las Lomas in July 2008. As I moved intellectually from suicide to psychiatry, my identity categories—Maya, indigenous, mestiza, indio—began to fall apart. Maya heritage, which had seemed so important at the outset of my work, quickly disappeared from my radar. None of the mental health professionals I worked with cared about Maya suicide goddesses or tourism development strategies, and neither did their patients. Identity, as a category of lived experience, remained an important part of my work. But other phenomena came to the fore. Psychiatry as a situated social practice. Interactions between doctors and patients. Health care reform. Invisible Beings. Through it all, three common threads emerged: madness, modernity, and coloniality, all of which will continue to appear throughout this book. In chapter 3, these three themes intersect within the walls of Las Lomas, as I consider the structure and practice of Mexican politics and psychiatry within its wards.

3 · MAKING THE MATRIX

El peor enemigo de un mexicano, es otro mexicano.

A Mexican's worst enemy is another Mexican.

—Mexican proverb

POLITICS AND BEDFELLOWS

It was 2008 in Valladolid, a small city in the eastern part of the state. I was conducting research on suicide and teaching at Universidad de Oriente (UNO) as a visiting professor when I was invited by one of my students, Fany, to a birthday party. She was an older student, a widow in her forties who had decided to return to school and pursue a degree in Maya language and culture when UNO first opened its doors in 2007. She had worked as a nurse for many years, and her late husband had practiced medicine in Valladolid. She still maintained close ties with the local community of health workers. Over lunch, the subject got around to the large new public hospital under construction in Merida. It was a huge, postmodern building, gleaming white, full of glass, high ceilings, and empty spaces. The facility, constructed with health department funding as a facility for patients with Seguro Popular, was a high-specialty hospital. Situated in a newer, affluent neighborhood directly across the street from a new private hospital, the high-specialty hospital was supposed to have opened in early 2008. Yet, when I saw it in May 2008, the facility was still under construction, and it was surrounded by buses and people holding signs in protest.

Back in Valladolid, Fany was telling me she had just gotten back from Merida. "I went with my sister-in-law and my cousin to protest the new hospital," she explained, "and we won! The administrators conceded to our demands."

"Oh?" I exclaimed, "I saw the buses outside. You were there? What happened?"

"It's the new specialty hospital," she explained. "They were going to bring doctors and nurses with advanced degrees from Cuba and other states in Mexico. It wasn't right! We went and protested, demanded the hospital hire just like the other ones: only people from Yucatan, and preference given to family members who work in the system."

For a moment, I was dumbfounded. Having grown up in the United States, I had never heard someone speaking of nepotism so brazenly. "What do you mean?"

Fany nodded enthusiastically. "So, let's say my sister-in-law's daughter studies nursing. If she applies for a job in the hospital, she will get it over someone who doesn't have any family in the system. It's how we do things. Positions are inherited. With this hospital, they were going to require advanced degrees for all the nurses who worked in it. Well, that would have cut out almost everyone in Yucatan, our nurses don't often have the opportunity to pursue advanced degrees. We weren't having it. So we went and protested. My sister-in-law, my cousin, and I, we camped out on the front lawn of the hospital! We slept right there on the grass. And we got them to concede! The hospital will be staffed by people from Yucatan. It won't require advanced degrees anymore."

I later found out Fany had been supporting more than 3,000 health worker union members—including doctors, nurses, and hospital administrators—who had participated in a twenty-four-hour work stoppage that affected more than 20,000 patients in eighteen hospitals throughout Merida (Boffil Gómez 2008). The health workers demanded the completion of the much-delayed construction project, the appointment of a different director, and guaranteed employment for 300 unionized health workers. The protesters had not simply camped out outside, but they took over the facilities in response to the announced hiring of 1,200 health workers from out of state (Proceso 2008).

As I came to learn, this story is neither unique nor remarkable—worker mobilization and institutionalized nepotism are an aspect of everyday life in Mexico, particularly when it comes to worker's unions (*sindicatos* or *gremios*). However, it unveils the complexity of political maneuvering in everyday life in ways that may be unexpected to readers unfamiliar with the Mexican context. The health worker mobilization illustrates what Nuijten (2003) called the "hope generating machine," the ways people form alliances and define tactics to compel the state to favorable action. At the same time, a sensible neoliberal subject might find the institutionalized nepotism that Fany assumes to be right and good to be morally repugnant, a stark contrast to the much-cherished value placed on meritocracy in the United States. As Gledhill (2004) notes, neoliberal reform has done much to dismantle the hope-generating machine, yet at the same time, the success of the health workers' mobilization in Merida demonstrates that the neoliberalization of Mexican society and the Mexican state remains incomplete—or, perhaps, that neoliberalism is not a uniform phenomenon, but one that necessarily adapts and changes according to local interests.

Fany's story illustrates the importance of relationships in the functioning of Mexican public institutions. Increasingly, more and more health workers—like Dr. Patrón, for instance—are hired on contract. They are given limited benefits, low pay, and are afforded no job security. However, most health workers are not on contract, but are unionized employees. In the twentieth century, during Mexico's seventy-one years of single-party rule, unions in Mexico were originally subsumed by the ruling party, the Partido Revolucionario Institucional (PRI), and so they were essentially part of the Mexican state, giving them significant power at the same time that it constrained them. With the democratic transition of 2000 came attempts at labor law reform, which resulted in some weakening, although the efforts to reform are largely at a standstill. However, the second decade of the twenty-first century witnessed serious challenges to the two most powerful unions in the country. The privatization of oil in Mexico and accompanying overhaul of the national petroleum company, Petroleos Mexicanos (PEMEX), worker benefits, as well as educational reform aimed at increasing teacher accountability (and the incarceration of teacher union president Elba Esther Gordillo in 2013) suggest that this weakening will continue. Although salaries in the Mexican health care institutions are low when compared to private-sector employment, the benefits, which include health care within the IMSS or ISSSTE insurance schemes, maternity leave, a generous pension, and home-purchasing assistance, are highly coveted. The broad acceptance of institutionalized nepotism is part of a culture in which relationships are far more important than merit in the administration of health institutions. This is an observation, not a moral judgment.

At Las Lomas, the complexity of official and nonofficial social relationships dictates the fortunes of everyone who works on its wards and, by extension, their patients. When I first met Dr. Juan Vasquez in 2007, I knew he was involved with a local suicide prevention organization, *La Vida es Bella*, and that he ran a suicide prevention program. I did not know that he had directed Las Lomas for twenty years, or that the reason he was in charge of Las Lomas's Emergency Room was that he had been exiled by the new (PAN-affiliated) hospital director to the most undesirable position in the hospital in an attempt by his political enemies to drive him out of the institution. I was also completely unaware of how Juan's situation was deeply intertwined with Yucatan's party politics.

Party politics affect professional as well as political careers in Mexico. For example, until 2016, Las Lomas fell under the purview of the Yucatan health secretariat. Governors serve six-year terms and have the right to appoint leadership positions throughout the state government. This includes the position of secretary of health, who in turn has the right to appoint directors at state public hospitals within the purview of the health secretariat. Before the year 2000, every governor of the state of Yucatan had been a member of the PRI party, which had held on to power at the federal level for seventy-one years. Before 2000, political futures depended on party politics, but—because only one party was ever in power—most power plays were made within the PRI rather than outside it. When I met him, Juan's personal political views were fairly independent, but he had been able to navigate the internal party politics of PRI well enough to retain his position as director of Las Lomas for twenty years.

The election of the opposition PAN (Partido de Acción Nacional) party to the governor's seat in Yucatan in 2001, following the 2000 federal election, was the first change in party at both the state and federal levels in seventy-one years. Even if there is no change in party lines, the people in positions of leadership—hospital directors, public health offices, municipal services—frequently rotate in and out of office every three (for municipal positions) to six (for state positions) years. Suddenly, the expected turnover and adjustment of leadership as one governor left office and another entered it became unpredictable. Juan found himself relegated to the emergency room of the institution he had built. His beloved suicide prevention program was closed down. In the six years that followed, Juan focused on his private practice, teaching, research, a weekly newspaper column, and his work with the local NGO *La Vida es Bella*, which took over the suicide prevention hotline. He made himself comfortable—he purchased an air conditioning unit for the emergency room with his own money and had it installed, brought a laptop and a wireless internet card, and spent his time between patients writing. A few years later, his former student, Dr. Tun, returned from an extended absence in Mexico City and joined him in the emergency room.

However, when the governor's seat went from PAN back to PRI, the old director was replaced with a more sympathetic ally. When I moved to Merida in June 2008, Juan had been given an office and a secretary, and the suicide prevention group was meeting once again. Juan still refers to his time in the emergency room as his *castigo* (his punishment) and the six-year dormancy of the suicide prevention program as criminal. By summer of 2008, when I joined La Esperanza, the program was well on its way to recovering its former robustness: all patients who were committed following suicide attempts were enrolled in La Esperanza and attended three inpatient group therapy sessions a week for the duration of their hospital stay. Every Thursday, an additional session was held for both inpatients and those who had previously been committed following suicide attempts. In 2008, Dr. Tun, who remained in the emergency room, was also an active participant. Every Thursday morning the room would fill, music would play, and when Juan entered, the room would erupt.

Over the six months I regularly attended La Esperanza meetings, I saw the emergence of a community and a free community resource. Between January 2008 and August 2017, 29,668 patients had participated in the program, many remaining involved in group activities over several years.[1] Over time, the group—mostly driven by former patients volunteering their time—expanded into other outreach activities, such as community theater performances in local schools and a weekly local radio show focused on suicide prevention. Although Juan can and does prescribe pharmaceutical treatment to his patients, the program's orientation is psychodynamic and consistent with Frommian psychology, which is focused on individual and group therapy as well as attentive to social context. During La Esperanza's six-year absence, patients who were committed following suicide attempts did not benefit from any program aimed at addressing the compounding social factors that frequently lead to suicide and suicide attempts (Reyes-Foster 2013b).

Mexico once again held state and federal elections in the summer of 2012, and this time Juan was not so lucky: the PRI party won again, and the new hospital director was not someone he got along with. By 2013, this directly affected me. When I returned to Las Lomas and met with the new hospital director, I was politely but firmly informed that I could no longer carry out research there. Although the director, Dr. Pasos, never explicitly said my permission to work in the hospital was revoked because of my relationship to Juan, Juan himself and several other friends and colleagues at Las Lomas believed that this was the case. Later on, when Dr. Tun and I met for coffee, she chided me—"You should have told me that you were going to meet him! I'm friends with him. I could have gotten you in."[2]

There is more to the story of Dr. Pasos and the end of my work at Las Lomas that illustrates the changing interpersonal dynamics interwoven in the everyday functioning of the psychiatric institution. In 2013, when I first arrived in Yucatan, I emailed Dr. Pasos at the generic Las Lomas director's email address and requested a meeting. The meeting was granted, and I arrived at Las Lomas on a muggy June morning at the scheduled time. When I was admitted into the director's office, I was met by a woman who simply introduced herself as Irma Gonzalez. Dr. Pasos was nowhere in sight. I took Irma to be Las Lomas's subdirector, because I knew from past experience that occasionally the hospital subdirector would take on these kinds of meetings in the director's stead. During my meeting with Irma, I explained the purpose of my research and handed her my IRB documentation. She took notes in a notebook, asked questions about what resources and personnel I would need to carry out my research, and told me Dr. Pasos would be in touch. A few days later, I received an email written by her from Dr. Pasos's personal email address, asking me to come in for another meeting. This time, Dr. Pasos was present. When I came in to the meeting, Dr. Pasos introduced Irma as Las Lomas's "codirector." At this meeting, Dr. Pasos informed me that I could no longer carry out research at Las Lomas.

As I was leaving the hospital, I passed by Yovana, Juan's secretary. She asked me how it went, and I told her.

"Did you meet Irma?" she asked.

"You mean the codirector?" I asked.

She rolled her eyes. "Yeah. The 'codirector.'"

Yovana explained what I had come to suspect: the hospital had no "codirector." Irma was Dr. Pasos's romantic partner, and she assisted him in all of his work, but she was not on the hospital payroll nor legally authorized to do any of the work she did, which included answering his emails and meeting with people like me.

Everyone at Las Lomas knew about Irma, yet she continued to assist Dr. Pasos for nearly two more years, until he resigned from his position.

These examples—the hospital workers' mobilization in support of institutional nepotism and regional favoritism, the suspension of the suicide prevention program out of what appears to be sheer spite, and the sudden revocation of access to my field site—illustrate the ways policy and interpersonal relationships constitute political reality in the Yucatecan state, albeit in different ways. Each example illustrates the role of alliances and personal networks in the functioning of the state. In the case of the workers' mobilization, Fany and her family members recognized that they shared a common interest with the workers in Merida toward maintaining the status quo. They were, in fact, resisting the neoliberalization of Mexican public medicine, which sees the health care workers' demands as inconvenient, expensive, and a violation of the ethos of meritocracy. For Juan and La Esperanza, which had been able to function under the old status quo of single-party rule, the much-celebrated democratic transition of party rule proved bitter. Finally, my own association with my primary collaborator and field mentor made me inherently suspect to the new hospital administrator, who, as an outsider, had his own agenda. Social realities do not necessarily or always fall into the category of "corruption" as it is generally understood, but they present violations of Western sensibilities of good governance. More importantly, they exemplify the interweaving of politics, bureaucracy, and relationships.

"EVERYBODY DOES IT"

The emergency room at Las Lomas is universally disliked by the medical staff, particularly the doctors and residents. With an unpredictable flow of patients, oftentimes slow, it affords few learning opportunities for eager residents and no opportunity for continuity of care for the attending psychiatrist. When one thinks of a psychiatric emergency, one might think of very dramatic events: a patient in the midst of a psychotic break, acting in a manner consistent with imaginaries of madness of the Global North, babbling incoherently, acting violent, in need of physical restraint. Most of the time, however, patients seeking emergency care do not arrive by ambulance in the throngs of psychosis. They walk in, accompanied by their family members. Dr. Daniel Patrón was the shift physician in charge of the day shift at Las Lomas in 2012, when I was conducting my research in the emergency room. Dr. Patrón was a contract physician—the equivalent of an academic adjunct in the United States—and was working in the emergency room while he waited for a permanent job opportunity to come along. He was from Mexico City, and he and his wife had moved to Yucatan to pursue their medical careers; he was an outgoing man with light skin, wire-rimmed glasses, and a mop of thick dark hair.

The importance of family support in the well-being of mentally ill patients cannot be understated. By the same token, family members who are primary caretakers face numerous challenges in navigating Mexico's complex medical system, particularly when it comes to accessing needed care and medications. Families meet these challenges through a variety of creative means, many of which contribute to the overall dysfunction of the medical systems themselves. The story of Don Gustavo, an elderly patient who arrived at the emergency room in July 2012, provides a case in point.

Don Gustavo was from a rural community near the gulf coast of Yucatan, about a two-hour drive from Las Lomas. He came to the emergency room accompanied by his wife, two daughters, and an adult granddaughter. His wife was a mestiza, but his daughters and granddaughter did not wear huipil. Don Gustavo wore grey slacks, a clean but yellowed guayabera, and a baseball hat. His granddaughter held his arm as he walked. On this day, Dr. Patrón was supervising Ana, an advanced psychiatry resident, and Daniela, a first-year psychiatry resident. As we will see in the following exchange, both residents participated in interviewing Don Gustavo and his family. Don Gustavo's wife explained that he was experiencing worsening symptoms of dementia. The medication he had was not helping him, and she wanted the doctors to give him a medication that could provide relief from the worst of his symptoms—sleeplessness, aggressiveness, and visual hallucinations. After assessing Don Gustavo's state of mind, asking questions of orientation (by assessing whether Don Gustavo could answer questions about his identity and location in space and time, discussed in chapters 4 and 5) and confirming he was not oriented in space or time, Dr. Patrón looked at the medication on the script and shook his head. "This isn't the medicine I would recommend for his condition," he started.

"We know! That's what they told us when we got it," his wife interrupted, "but *El Seguro* [IMSS] didn't have the medication they wanted to give him, so they sent him home with this."

Don Gustavo's granddaughter spoke up. "The problem is IMSS. They prescribe medication in their hospital but then the IMSS pharmacy never has it in stock." Heads nodded in agreement—on both sides of the room—as Dr. Patrón let out a frustrated "hmm" in acknowledgment.

Don Gustavo's enrollment in IMSS should have been a blessing to his family. Under IMSS (described more fully in chapter 4) Don Gustavo should have been receiving regular, high-quality medical care and prescriptions free of charge, but the institution has been in crisis for many years and medication shortages and stockouts are commonplace. IMSS beneficiaries can take their prescriptions and purchase medication out-of-pocket at private pharmacies, but Don Gustavo's family did not have the financial means to do so.

Ana, Dr. Patrón's senior resident, proposed an alternative. "Why don't you enroll him in Seguro Popular?" referring to the newer health care scheme for the uninsured, which operates its own pharmacy networks and experiences fewer shortages.

Dr. Patrón started shaking his head almost as soon as she said it. Don Gustavo's oldest daughter, a woman in her fifties, looked back and forth between Ana and Dr. Patrón. Ana briefly nodded at Daniela, a first-year resident who was also in the room, and Daniela took over the interview, asking the family about Don Gustavo's sleeping habits and diet, as Ana and Dr. Patrón stepped away from the desk but stood within earshot of Don Gustavo and his family. I continued to sit at Dr. Patrón's desk, scribbling notes on the conversation as quickly as I could:

> Ana is suggesting that Patrón recommend that the family enroll Don Gustavo in Seguro Popular, because they would be able to access the medication free of cost. Patrón vehemently disagrees, noting that it would be unethical for them to suggest it because it is illegal to double up on state insurance and Don Gustavo is already enrolled in IMSS. Ana retorts that "everyone does it," and the ethical thing is for Don Gustavo to get the medication he needs. Daniela has run out of questions and Don Gustavo and his family sit silently, staring at the desk, waiting for Patrón and Ana to return. (Field notes, July 2012)

Without coming to an agreement, Ana and Dr. Patrón returned to the consultation desk. Dr. Patrón sat down at his chair and Ana stood next to him. Ana addressed the family first.

ANA: Look, the ideal thing for you to do is to enroll your husband in Seguro Popular.

DR. PATRÓN: Okay, we are going to take you off all of these medications. I am going to prescribe this one, it's called Sapex and it's for sleeping. This one is Seroquel and it's for him to not see things anymore. [He writes the prescription and hands it to them]. To fill them through El Seguro you will have to take them back to the IMSS hospital and have an IMSS prescription written for them. Then you can fill them at the IMSS pharmacy at no cost, provided they have them. Or you can buy them out of pocket.

DAUGHTER: So do you recommend we enroll my father in Seguro Popular?

DR. PATRÓN: *La doctora* [gesturing toward Ana] suggests you enroll him in Seguro Popular so he gets his medication filled there. But in either case take him to the Family Medicine Office so that he has blood work done, because you all need to know how he is doing.

Although we do not know whether Don Gustavo's family followed Ana's advice, Dr. Patrón's description of what Don Gustavo's family would have to do to obtain the medication he prescribed is extremely difficult: *Take [the prescription] back to the IMSS hospital and have an IMSS prescription written for them.* (The IMSS hospital is at least two bus rides away from Las Lomas in a major metropolitan area unfamiliar to the family. The family will then have to wait to have the Las Lomas script converted into an IMSS script—which may require an additional evaluation by an IMSS doctor and a longer wait time, assuming they are willing to see him without an appointment, which usually needs to be made several weeks in advance.) *Then you can fill them at the IMSS pharmacy at no cost, provided they have them.* (This effort may be for naught if the medication is out of stock, which is the reason the family came to Las Lomas in the first place.) *Or you can buy them out of pocket.* (This would be logistically easiest, but the costliest solution for the family, even if they had the financial means.) The task is gargantuan, especially when trying to carry it out using public transportation with a frail and confused old man in tow. Dr. Patrón, without conceding that Ana is right, did not try to dissuade the family from enrolling in Seguro Popular, even though he believes this is an unethical abuse of the medical system. Despite his personal objection to the practice of doubling up on insurance, he recognized the structural obstacles the family faced in accessing health care when they did not.

This exchange illustrates a major conundrum faced by medical practitioners throughout Mexico. The disagreement between Ana, an advanced psychiatry resident on the cusp of finishing her specialization, and Dr. Patrón, a practicing psychiatrist on contract at Las Lomas, is probably one that takes place among all doctors currently trying to practice medicine in Mexico. Is it wrong for patients who cannot obtain necessary treatment under one health care scheme (IMSS) to illegally sign up to receive care under another (Seguro Popular)? The medication shortages that prompted Don Gustavo's family to walk into the psychiatric emergency room, even though they have access to free medical care and, were it available, free medication, exemplify the inadequacies of the state medical systems. The family faces a moral dilemma. Given that the state has failed Don Gustavo by not having stock of the medication to which he is legally entitled and has a prescription, is Don Gustavo's family justified in obtaining the medication from another medical scheme, although it would mean breaking the law and straining the system? Does Don Gustavo's family owe compliance to the state if it fails to uphold its end of the social contract?

Moral conundrums aside, before a cross-referencing program was developed in 2014, Mexican citizens enrolled in IMSS or ISSSTE could and frequently did also enroll in Seguro Popular. Although official figures are unavailable, in January 2016 the health secretary of the state of Zacatecas announced that 82,000 IMSS and ISSSTE enrollees were also enrolled in Seguro Popular and would be de-enrolled when their three-year policies expired (Salinas 2016).[3] During my research period at Las Lomas (2008–2013), it was remarkably easy to enroll in Seguro Popular, as double enrollments could be detected only when enrollment databases were compared to one another, and this was not regularly done. When duplicates were found, patients did not immediately lose their coverage. While some, like Dr. Patrón, may argue that such actions constitute an abuse of the medical system posing long-term risk to the viability of the program, others, like Ana, argue that people must do what they can to survive when the state fails to meet its responsibilities toward its citizens. Later, when Dr. Patrón and I discussed his views of doubling on up on insurance care, he explained that to him, enrolling in dual insurance was a form of "cheating" the system (*hacer trampa*). If "everyone" doubles up on insurance, he reasoned, how would the new system ever work fairly or sustainably? *This is the problem with Mexicans,* he and others explained when we talked about the shortcomings of the Mexican health care systems and other social programs; *we are always looking out for ourselves and not thinking about the impact of our actions on society.* Shaking his head in dismay, Dr. Patrón stated an adage I have heard many times before: *El peor enemigo de un mexicano es otro mexicano* (A Mexican's worst enemy is another Mexican).

This sentiment—that actions motivated by self-interest are an indelible and harmful part of Mexican-ness—has a long history. In *The Labyrinth of Solitude* ([1950] 1993), Octavio Paz argues that Mexican people share an inherent distrust that leads them to undermine one another. He writes, "Para el mexicano, la vida es una posibilidad de chingar o de ser chingado" (For the Mexican, life is the possibility of fucking or getting fucked) (88). As I will discuss, this fatalist perspective is often bemoaned in public conversations about role of culture in Mexico's perceived slowness to develop into a fully "modern" state (Mayer-Serra 2014). It also has the effect of depoliticizing serious structural shortcomings of the Mexican state and political governance in the name of "culture" and "corruption."

Conversations about the ethics of doubling up on insurance and its effects on Mexican society reflect a broader societal concern with the intermingled problems of governance, corruption, and the social contract in the context of the Mexican state. For people like Ana, doubling up on insurance is essentially a weapon of the weak (Scott 1985), a tactic by which citizens use the state in a piecemeal fashion to compensate for its deficiencies. For people like Dr. Patrón, it represents everything wrong with Mexican society. At heart is a tense and combative relationship between the Mexican state and the Mexican people. The state is seen as a source of support but also a source of chaos (Gledhill 2004).

For progressive Mexicans, corruption—be it in the form of systemic corruption in the Mexican state or in the form of small-scale abuses of the system—remains the single most important obstacle to modernization. For decades, Mexican economists, historians, and political scientists have spilled frustrated ink over what they perceive to be the single greatest obstacle to Mexican modernity. In 2014, President Enrique Peña Nieto publicly stated that Mexico was plagued by a "culture of corruption" (Rubí 2014). International relations expert and public intellectual Carlos Elizondo Mayer-Serra (2014) published a scathing critique of Peña Nieto's statement in the national daily *Excelsior*: "If we accept that corruption is cultural, we would have to accept that the modernization of our country is not possible in the short term. Things are how they are because we are how we are. There is no need for reform. If the government, shielded by the idea that this is a cultural phenomenon, is tolerant of corruption, it runs the risk of failing in transforming the country." Mayer-Serra cannot accept corruption as somehow part of Mexico's "culture." While this quotation may reflect overly simplistic understandings of nearly every concept mentioned ("culture," "corruption," "Mexico," "modern"), Mayer-Serra also implies that Mexico is somehow not "modern."

As I stated at the outset of this book, a concern with modernity and modernizing is at the forefront of the Mexican state's conversation with itself in the twenty-first century, as it has been since independence from Spain in 1821. "Modernity" always seems to be an elusive goal, a struggle, something just beyond the nation's reach. This view of modernity and its relationship to culture and corruption is not unique to Mexico, but it can be found throughout Latin America (Gledhill 2004; Nuijten 2003). Yet, as I argue in chapter 1, what modernity *is* cannot be assumed a priori. Modernity(ies) are processes and products—capitalism, representative democracy, scientific epistemology—of historical events constituted by the colonial matrix of power (Quijano 1992; Rivera Cusicanqui 2010; Mignolo 2011; Grosfoguel 2011a, 2011b). As anthropologists of corruption have argued (Gupta 1995; Gledhill 2004; Nuijten and Anders 2007; Smith 2007), practices indexed as "corrupt" are frequently understood in the context of modernist discourses of "development," but this view reduces their social complexity to a problem in need of a solution (Gledhill 2004, 173–174). An anthropological perspective demands these practices be understood as products of their own social context. As Smith (2007) and others have shown, everyday practices coproduce corruption, yet they are frequently necessary for everyday survival. Corruption at once responds to inequality and perpetuates it. Doubling up on IMSS and Seguro Popular may undermine the national strategy of universal health care (thus perpetuating inequality), but the alternative is doing without essential and necessary care and medications.

Mexico's newspapers are full of editorials by prominent public intellectuals like Mayer-Serra, who argue that corruption is holding the nation back from fulfilling its mandate to modernize, assuming "modern" to be synonymous with an economic and bureaucratic efficiency that is possible only when nobody "cheats" (Reyes Heroles 2001, 2015; Mayer-Serra 2014). In other words, the politician who abuses his government position to embezzle money from the state is engaged in the same kind of behavior as Don Gustavo's family doubling up on insurance or families who abandon their relatives at the hospital—the difference is merely one of scale. For them, it is *all* corruption. However, there are other viewpoints. For example, historian Guillermo Marín (2001) makes a different argument. Drawing on Guillermo Bonfil Batalla's classic text, *Mexico Profundo* (1987), Marín argues that corruption is a "strategy of cultural resistance of the peoples who conform . . . Deep Mexico" (14), referring to Bonfil Batalla's argument that Mexican culture, and by consequence the Mexican state, is characterized by a systematic negation and suppression of its indigenous origins and contemporary indigenous cultures.

In Bonfil Batalla's and Marín's view, the people who make up "Deep Mexico" are Mexico's poor and indigenous peoples. Marín's argument is explicitly decolonial (1987, 11). Pointing out that the invasion, domination, and legalized exploitation of the Americas, Asia, and Africa is at the foundation of the wealth of the powerful nations of the Global North, Marín notes that allegedly endemic corruption in former colonies has served the interests of former colonizers, who have profited from the corrupt practices of elites at the same time as they have given themselves a moralizing upper hand. "We have imported these judgments about the incorruptibility of laws, institutions, and authorities, originating in colonizing countries or the so-called first world, and, as always, we have clumsily and superficially tried to apply them to our own reality . . . could we suppose that, if corruption has existed for so long among us, that it is not a 'terrible evil,' as we have always believed? . . . [could it be that] corruption has been something 'good' for the survival of our civilization and our identity?" (10–11). Marín thus differentiates between the kinds of corrupt practices of elites and the actions of people in everyday life, for whom corruption (in the form of bribery, tips, stealth, subterfuge, petty theft, opportunism, etc.) is not merely a weapon of the weak, but a tactic of cultural survival. Marín and others (Nieto 2013) contend that a tactic such as doubling up on insurance can be understood not only as a tactic of resistance or weapon of the weak, but as engaging in a broadly accepted rejection of the modern Mexican state.

Others have gone as far as to argue that corruption is such an indelible part of Mexican institutions that these would likely crumble in the face of real attempts at reform (Morris 1991). U.S. political scientist Stephen Morris (2011, 2009, 1991) argues that what scholars and politicians in Mexico refer to as "corruption" is in fact a wide range of practices that emerge as a response to the state's own policy failings. At the heart of Mexico's struggle with corruption, he argues, "is a fundamental lack of legitimacy. Mexicans rarely trust the law, governmental institutions, or their politicians" (Morris 2011, 329). By engaging in activities considered to be forms of corruption, he argues, Mexicans reveal an anti-state, pro-society bias. This argument finds some echo in anthropological writings of corruption in other postcolonial societies.[4] Thus, it is possible to appreciate that what at first appears to be an instance of corruption can be read as another way by which actors on the ground use the medical institution's own inefficiencies for their own survival, such as, in this case, to obtain needed medications.

There are other ways by which ordinary people deploy tactics and use the state and its institutions to achieve their own goals.[5] Lina, introduced in more detail in chapter 4, was familiar with hospital protocols, successfully engaging in behaviors she knew would achieve a desired outcome. Lina behaved in ways that automatically trigger specific hospital responses. Self-injury would result in the use of restraints. Reporting suicidal ideation would delay her transfer out of the intensive care ward. When Dr. Tun, her attending physician, tried to minimize contact with Lina, believing that what she wanted was attention, Lina became so disruptive to the ward—crying, screaming, picking fights with other patients—she needed to be sedated. The hospital did not have a specific protocol to deal with a patient who knew how to get herself committed and medicated, and Dr. Tun, feeling that her hands were tied, frequently expressed feelings of frustration. This tactic is not unique to Lina or Las Lomas; psychiatric patients frequently discovered patterns of behavior that achieved certain results. Lina's background as a mental health care professional gave her an edge, but years of treatment and multiple hospitalizations likely provided her with an arsenal of tactics, echoing E. Summerson Carr's (2011) description of how therapeutic scripts are used and manipulated by patients and providers in a U.S. addiction treatment facility. But while patients deploy tactics in attempts to achieve their own goals, the greater strategies of political power that determine much of Las Lomas's administration affect doctors and patients in different ways. Of course, patients like Lina, who wish to be confined at Las Lomas, were rare; most patients I encountered felt victimized by the medical system, inside and outside of Las Lomas, and had no wish to be resident.

ANDREA

July 17, 2012, was a quiet day in the acute care ward. With some of her teaching responsibilities relieved with the start of the Mexican summer break, Dr. Tun seemed unusually relaxed. We had our usual heavy consultation docket—six names on the list, three of whom had been admitted overnight. One name stood out: Andrea M., and next to her name, the ICD F20.0 diagnosis (schizophrenia) was followed by the note, under the "comorbidity" column: *crónica*, meaning that Andrea had been designated as a permanently committed patient at Las Lomas and was not expected to be ever be released. This "comorbidity" designation seemed to counter the dominant anti-asylum discourse that I saw everywhere at Las Lomas. Until that point, the message I had been getting from doctors at Las Lomas was consistent with the neoliberal ideologies of the Global North: Las Lomas had made a definitive turn away from the asylum model of care decades ago. *Crónicos*, permanently committed patients, were a thing of the past.

There were not supposed to be any more chronic patients committed to Las Lomas. Although some sixty "chronic" patients continued to reside permanently in Las Lomas, and would likely live out the rest of their lives there, this was because they had been there before the hospital made the definitive turn to biomedicine and away from institutionalization. All these patients had been committed more than twenty years ago, most to the old Hospital Ayala prior to Las Lomas's construction in 1978. Alternative accommodations outside the hospital were not possible, and there truly appeared to be no other option for them. I knew some of these patients by sight or reputation: there was one older man who had been lobotomized in the 1960s; a woman who had developed an obsession with one of her professors in her first year of medical school and who continued to live in a state of delusion, convinced that her feelings were reciprocated. But my interactions with them were fleeting, my knowledge of them nothing more than anecdotes whispered by Las Lomas residents and staff. With the shift toward biomedical care associated with the construction and opening of Las Lomas in the 1970s, "crónicos" were supposed to become a thing of the past. But despite its modernist beginnings and commitment to deinstitutionalization, Las Lomas continued to have a reputation as a place for families to abandon their mentally ill or intellectually disabled relatives when they were unable to care for them. As my friend and colleague Juan Vasquez liked to say, there was a reason that the new psychiatric hospital had been built next to the city dump.

Against all logic and the hospital's own official stance, Andrea had been permanently committed fourteen months prior, in May 2011, although her file number revealed she had been in and out of Las Lomas for nearly ten years. Because Las Lomas did not adequately protect its patients from mosquitoes nor take any precautions to reduce the mosquito population, it was common for patients at Las Lomas to become infected with dengue and chikungunya, especially during the rainy season, which usually spans from June to August. In July 2012, Andrea was admitted into the acute care ward for further observation because of symptoms that indicated a possible dengue fever infection; otherwise I would have never come into contact with her. Dr. Tun shook her head in disapproval as she opened the case file. "There is a request from the municipality for *resguardo* [a legal term indicating the local police had requested Andrea be confined] here. She's probably the town drunk," she said, as she thumbed through it, "and they wanted to clean up the governor's town." According to the file, Andrea, a native of Dzemul (the same municipality that Ivonne Ortega, the outgoing governor, came from), had initially been brought to Las Lomas after arrest for public drunkenness, but sometime after her involuntary commitment, she was reassigned as a chronic patient.

Dr. Tun and Carolina began talking about how, despite the state's anti-asylum rhetoric, Las Lomas was still viewed as a zone of abandonment by local society and the Yucatecan state. "In 2005, when the state government expanded the State Hospital in Merida," Dr. Tun remembered, "the hospital literally sent us the indigent people who slept in its entrances. They put them in police trucks and they arrived at Las Lomas, bags and all."

"And did they stay?" I asked.

"Yes," she answered sardonically, "but without their bags."

Andrea's case and Dr. Tun's retelling of the indigents brought to Las Lomas from the General Hospital are reminiscent of other stories of social abandonment explored by anthropologists over the years (Biehl 2005; Marrow and Luhrmann 2012; Varley 2016). The story also brings into question the role of institutionalization in state policy, particularly toward the homeless. There are few data on homelessness in Yucatan. While homelessness and indigency have been studied locally by the municipal government of Merida (*Diario de Yucatan* 2016, 2017), there is no available evidence of the psychiatric hospital being systematically or officially used to "clean up the streets." Such studies have suggested that Merida's indigent population is mostly comprised of elderly people who have family members unwilling to care for them. These studies have also found that many of Merida's indigent people are not homeless. However, in my time at Las Lomas, I met several patients who had experienced periods of homelessness or who had resorted to panhandling or sex work as a means of survival. I also met patients who, while not homeless, were identified in their local communities as "the town drunk" or "the town lunatic" and were targeted for abuse by other community members. It was not unusual for these patients to be judicially committed (as the result of an arrest) following an altercation with either community members who antagonized them or the local authorities. Looking through Andrea's file, this appeared to be the case; she had been arrested for public drunkenness and brought to Las Lomas. However, in other ways, Andrea's story was an aberration, as it was not normal for one of these patients to be permanently committed. Usually, the hospital staff makes a concerted effort to move patients through and out of the institution.

Patients and hospital staff alike navigate Las Lomas according to their own degrees of agency, determined greatly by the kinds of relationships they form with one another and the institution. In chapter 2, I described the emergence of Zona del Estar, a bridge between zones of being and nonbeing, as a way of understanding the temporality of madness in Las Lomas. In the following chapters, I take that conceptual construct and explore what it means in practice. In the Zona del Estar, sanity and madness intersect with social structure. It is a space for the deployment of tactics that shape everyday life, often in opposition to existing state strategies seeking to do the same. In this chapter, I explore the ways in which competing actors and institutions with varying degrees of agency interact and intersect with the Mexican and Yucatecan states in the context of Las Lomas. I show how actors on the ground deploy a variety of tactics in response to various state strategies to further particular interests. In deploying these tactics, actors affect other actors and groups of actors who themselves are also seeking to further their own interests. I illustrate how these actions, reactions, and interactions create a complex web of social processes against the backdrop of the state. This web, I argue, is constitutive of the colonial matrix of power.

The colonial matrix of power as originally described by Quijano (2000) refers to the coming together of various realms—authority, sexuality, labor, and subjectivity—to affect all aspects of life in modernity. While others have critiqued this conceptual framework as too limiting (it conflates sexuality with gender, for instance), the notion that the colonial matrix of power is constituted through the interweaving of colonial logics in different aspects of life remains useful, particularly when trying to understand the persistence of coloniality and colonial power relations even after attempts are made to decolonize, such as during the Mexican Revolution. The colonial matrix of power is persistent in large part because of the capillary nature of power (Foucault 1972): in other words, it operates and is constituted in deep but microscopic ways, in small-scale actions and interactions as well as in social structure.

The relationship between madness, modernity, and coloniality in the Zona del Estar can be understood by exploring the strategies and tactics of everyday life at Las Lomas. I do this in the following way. First, I explore cases of social abandonment, the institution's response, and their ultimate outcome. Second, I describe the ways in which patients, with the willing and sometimes unwilling help of psychiatrists, use the institution for their own purposes. In each case we see a strategy, devised structurally by the state, and an opposing tactic that undermines it. The state rejects the asylum model, but people continue to abandon their unwanted family members there. The government creates a health care plan for the uninsured, but because of the shortcomings of the other health care system, people enroll in both public health care plans. Political appointments determine hospital leadership, but personal rivalries and vendettas undermine the functioning of the institution.

In each instance I describe in this chapter, I identify different social processes taking place inside the constraints of the medical institution. These processes entail different modes of navigating what is at times an unwieldy and uncompromising bureaucracy. In this chapter, I do not examine bureaucracy as a defined object of study; rather, bureaucracy presents a structural backdrop, a setting in which the practices and interactions I discuss occur. Bureaucracy limits and defines the scope of action, but it is not, in this instance, a defined actor or entity.[6] I also explore the myriad ways in which actors deploy tactics that reveal the complexity of life and everyday functioning inside Mexican public health institutions, and the ways actors engage and create processes constitutive of the colonial matrix of power.

Something was not right with Andrea's file, something that suggested maybe she was not just a social undesirable who had been abandoned in Las Lomas's wards. She was officially diagnosed with schizophrenia, yet she was not taking any medications, and she was not symptomatic. Her case file was missing pages of notes, including her medical history and her history of admissions to the hospital, including the note that should have justified her status as a "crónica." When Dr. Tun interviewed Andrea, she denied ever hearing voices, saying simply that she had come to the hospital because of *nervios*, a common idiom of distress in Latin America (Guarnaccia, DeLaCancela, and Carrillo 1989). Andrea knew exactly how long she had been committed, and when she had last been given medication—March, several months earlier. Yet when Dr. Tun asked her whether she wanted to leave, Andrea smiled a close-mouthed, inscrutable smile before responding.

DR. TUN: Have you ever heard voices?
ANDREA: No.
DR. TUN: Why did you come to the hospital?
ANDREA: Nervios.
DR. TUN: Are you able to sleep at night?
ANDREA: Yes.
DR. TUN: With medication or without medication?
ANDREA: Without.
DR. TUN: How are you feeling? How is your pain?
ANDREA: I feel good, it's gone.
DR. TUN: Do you feel you have the energy to run? To shout?
ANDREA: [Chuckles] yes.
DR. TUN: So what do you do all day, Andrea? In your ward?
ANDREA: Well, I go to occupational therapy, then I come back.
DR. TUN: It would be good for you to go to a shelter, don't you think? So instead of living in the hospital you could live in a shelter, in a home?
ANDREA: That would be good.
DR. TUN: Of course, you would have a better life. You would be able to wear your own clothing, whatever you like.
ANDREA: Yes.
DR. TUN: We're going to suggest it, to have you transferred to a shelter. Hopefully I won't get in trouble!
ANDREA: [Smiles] yes.

The fact that Andrea was committed with a schizophrenia diagnosis but was completely unmedicated profoundly bothered Dr. Tun. She remarked on it the first time Andrea's file landed on her desk, and each day she met with her over the next few days. Hence, during the interview and over Andrea's three-day stay in the acute care ward, she repeatedly asked Andrea questions about symptoms and medication. The interview was the last interview Dr. Tun held with Andrea—Andrea recovered from her fever, and the fears of dengue turned out to be unfounded. She went back to her ward with a promise from Dr. Tun that she would try to get her transferred to a long-term women's shelter. I never saw her again. This exchange suggests Dr. Tun's relative powerlessness regarding Andrea's future. Indeed, despite her irritation, Dr. Tun's options were limited. She was not Andrea's attending physician—that was a doctor in another ward—so she personally could not order her release nor have her transferred to a different facility. Furthermore, a reading of her incomplete file revealed that the hospital administration was aware of her presence at Las Lomas and her chronic designation.

Dr. Tun could have reported Andrea's case to Yucatan Comisión de Derechos Humanos del Estado de Yucatan (CODHEY),[7] a governmental agency dedicated to investigating allegations of human rights abuses throughout the state, but she did not. It is possible that she, like others who were complicit even if not directly benefiting from this irregular arrangement, simply did not have the political stomach to file a complaint that would have implicated the director of Las Lomas. Moreover, Yucatan's election had just taken place on July 2, and governor Ivonne Ortega was effectively on her way out. Shortly after I returned to the United States, Andrea was released from Las Lomas and ostensibly returned home to Dzemul. To the best of my knowledge, she did not return to Las Lomas.

Neither Dr. Tun nor I knew why Andrea was committed. We speculated that Andrea's commitment may have been a favor: Las Lomas kept an unruly individual off the streets of the governor's quiet town, and the institution gained some kind of public benefit. I do not know what Andrea thought of her situation—I did not have the opportunity to speak personally with her, and she was always guarded during her conversations with Dr. Tun. She seemed amenable to Dr. Tun's suggestion that she be transferred to a shelter, but what she really thought and felt remains a mystery. During my research in Las Lomas, I met several patients who had been abandoned at Las Lomas, though in nearly all instances the patients were eventually transferred elsewhere.

ABANDONED IN THE PSYCHIATRIC WARD

In 2008, Vannia was committed to Las Lomas following a suicide attempt, and so I met her while I was conducting my research on suicide prevention. A mother of two from a working-class neighborhood in Merida, Vannia had escaped an abusive spouse and moved with her children to a shelter, but her former spouse continued to abuse and harass her. This eventually led to her suicide attempt at the shelter, at which time her children were taken by the state and moved to a state children's center. They were homeless, and Vannia had no relatives willing to help. Due to her suicide attempt and subsequent commitment, Vannia lost her place at the shelter. When she first arrived at Las Lomas, she was treated for depression and attended La Esperanza group therapy sessions three times a week. As the weeks and months went by, I saw other patients come and go, and yet Vannia stayed. Every time I saw her in group therapy she would sit, smiling, listening, and when it was her turn, she would speak briefly, invariably about wanting to get better so that she could be reunited with her children.

Vannia was committed to Las Lomas around the time I started my field research in June 2008. Several situations complicated Vannia's case. She had no family and no home. Because of microcephaly, she had an abnormally small head and suffered from moderate intellectual disability, meaning she could not live on her own. Without a social network of support, her options were limited. She was still committed when I left in December 2008, though her social worker had finally found a shelter to which she could be transferred. She had also been able to visit her children at the children's center facility, although it was unlikely they would ever be permanently reunited. Unlike Andrea, whose extended commitment appeared to be the result of unethical and possibly illicit dealing, Vannia's extended stay appears to be related to her lack of a social safety net. In other words, this was a problem of abandonment.

In their investigations into the living conditions of people suffering from mental illness or living with disabilities in Mexican institutions, Disabilities Rights International (MDRI 2000; DRI 2011, 2015) has identified the problem of abandonment as a significant challenge to the rights of people with disabilities and mental illness in Mexican society. *Los abandonados* (the abandoned) are people who cannot live independently and have no one to care for them in the community. DRI documented thousands of cases across twenty facilities in Central Mexico of people with mental illnesses and disabilities who were left to languish in psychiatric institutions like Las Lomas for years. In some places, people will arrive at a psychiatric facility for acute treatment, and depending on the facility, may be referred to a network of residential shelters. This was Vannia's case. However, DRI notes that even these residential shelters are locked facilities, and residents are segregated into these shelters, away from local communities, for the long term. The United Nations Convention on the Rights of People with Disabilities (CRPD), the creation of which Mexico played a pivotal role, explicitly identifies long-term institutionalization as a violation of the right of all people with disabilities "to live in the community with choices equal to others" (United Nations 2006, Article 19). In my research at Las Lomas, my interlocutors frequently expressed concern and frustration with patients they suspected were being abandoned. The hospital social workers were usually, but not always, able to locate family members and persuade them to retrieve their loved ones, usually by facilitating access to the few community resources available. Nevertheless, patient abandonment remained a challenge and concern at Las Lomas.

In May 2012, I met Doña Isabel, an elderly woman in her eighties. She arrived overnight at Las Lomas, and she refused to meet with Dr. Tun on her first morning in the intensive care unit. Doña Isabel's patient file was thick—this was not her first visit to Las Lomas—but her last hospital stay had taken place in 2002, ten years prior. She scowled at Dr. Tun as she tried to conduct an initial interview during consultation. Dr. Tun would ask her a question, and Doña Isabel would give either single-word answers or would refuse to answer.

"You seem angry," Dr. Tun finally said, "Are you angry at someone?"

"No."

"Are you sure? Because you seem very angry."

"Angry?" Doña Isabel raised her thin arms from her wheelchair, and flashed us a toothless smile, "Look at me, I'm happy, I'm dancing!" she exclaimed, as she swayed her arms back and forth.

Dr. Tun stopped pressing the matter of Doña Isabel's anger. The conversation continued, and Dr. Tun asked Doña Isabel the same question she asked every patient on their first interview: "Why are you here?"

Doña Isabel's scowl deepened. "¡Por boba! [Because I was gullible!]"[8]

The conversation continued, as Doña Isabel sat, sullen and scowling in her wheelchair. According to her file, she had been diagnosed with schizophrenia and committed at Las Lomas many years ago; however, she had not been treated at Las Lomas for over a decade. The file did not contain important information about the circumstances that had brought her to Las Lomas this time: the emergency room admission note simply stated she had been dropped off by a family member, but no reason was given. Doña Isabel did not appear to be psychotic. She wore a plastic wristband from an all-inclusive resort on the Riviera Maya—only recently, she had been at an expensive hotel. Her speech and demeanor suggested she came from one of Yucatan's elite or upper middle classes. And yet she was committed to Las Lomas for reasons that were not entirely clear to Dr. Tun, as Doña Isabel's hostility made her difficult to interview. We did know this was her third day at Las Lomas, and she had no visitors. No family members came to request information about her condition. As far as we could tell, she had simply been left here.

As I left for the day, something—maybe the sound of rubber sandals scraping against cement—made me turn around. Doña Isabel was shuffling after me. Although she had been brought in for consultation in a wheelchair that morning, Doña Isabel apparently still had some mobility. She followed me out the unit doors, and came toward me, a few steps down the path leading to the main administrative building. I faced her and waited for her to catch up to me. Behind her, a nurse was slowly making his way toward us. I was wearing a blouse patterned after a huipil, a common textile worn by local women. This one was particularly colorful, with brightly colored embroidered flowers laid in a thick pattern around the square collar. Doña Isabel reached out and fingered the embroidery admiringly, the way only people who know how to embroider do.

"It's beautiful," she murmured.

"Thank you," I said.

Before I could say another word, the nurse reached us and gently touched her arm. Doña Isabel smiled at me and let him lead her back to the ward.

The next morning, I was late arriving at Las Lomas; the institution was two bus rides away from my home, and the buses were particularly full that morning. When I walked through the doors of the acute care ward unit, I found Doña Isabel, back in her wheelchair, sitting in the main entrance foyer directly in front of the door. Her arms were tied to the armrests with soft white strips of fabric, an IV drip connected to her arm. She dozed in her chair, her chin on her chest, snoring softly. As I came in, Dr. Tun and Carolina were busily writing up patient notes. They were between patients.

"Doña Isabel became dehydrated overnight," Dr. Tun explained when I asked about her, "so we had to put an IV in. She had to be restrained because she kept taking it out."

As she was talking, the door opened and Gladis, the head shift nurse came in. "Doña Isabel woke up and managed to take the IV out again, *doctora*."

Dr. Tun let out an exasperated sigh. "Give me one moment."

As soon as Gladis stepped out, Carolina shook her head. "Funny how she manages to do that."

Dr. Tun shook her head. "Yes. Funny," she said as she walked out.

I did not understand what was unspoken between them—although something clearly had—until many weeks later, after I had witnessed several similar exchanges. Dr. Tun's orientation as a psychiatrist was heavily influenced by Frommian psychoanalysis. She did not like to overmedicate her patients, and this frequently caused problems between her and the nursing staff. What was unspoken, as Dr. Tun and Carolina both explained in separate interviews, was their suspicion that Doña Isabel had been allowed to take her own IV out, with the purpose of getting Dr. Tun to authorize additional medication to keep Doña Isabel sedated and easier to manage.[9]

Without anyone to care enough about Doña Isabel, there was no one to know what might happen to her in the ward, or to advocate for her, to intervene if she was physically restrained or overmedicated, to note whether her symptoms improved or worsened. People like Doña Isabel must be managed, and without anyone to care what happens to her, she was particularly vulnerable to the ways in which the institution acted upon the bodies of the patients committed to its wards.

A few days after my encounter with Doña Isabel, I met Heidi. Heidi, just out of her teens, suffered from a moderate intellectual disability. She had been committed to Las Lomas in March and had been staying in the long-term care ward. She had returned to the acute ward following an altercation with another patient.

During the interview, Dr. Tun tried to elicit more information from Heidi.

DR. TUN: Heidi, who did you have a problem with?

HEIDI: Nobody. I want to go back to the other ward.

DR. TUN: Why do you want to go back to the other ward? What do you like to do there?

HEIDI: I like to make art, and walk around the garden.

DR. TUN: Do you have any friends?

HEIDI: Yes.

DR. TUN: Don't worry, Heidi, you will go back to the other ward. I'm just trying to understand how you're doing. Have you had any visitors?

HEIDI: No.

DR. TUN: [With disbelief] really?

CAROLINA: [Reading over Heidi's file.] She's right. She has not had any visitors.

DR. TUN: [Her expression changes, becomes softer.] Heidi, how have you been feeling? Have you been crying? Did you cry yesterday?

HEIDI: Yes. I miss my mother [her voice breaks, and she begins to cry].

DR. TUN: Okay, we will have the social worker locate your mother and see if we can get her to come visit.

CAROLINA: [She has continued reading over Heidi's file.] Dr. Tun, her mother is in Heaven.

HEIDI: She's in Heaven.

DR. TUN: Oh, I see. Who is supposed to be visiting you?

HEIDI: My sister.

DR. TUN: Okay Heidi. We will locate your sister so she can come see you. Now, I'm going to have the nurse take your vital signs, and if everything looks okay, I will send you back to the other ward, okay?

Heidi went back to the dormitory. Carolina continued looking over the file, shaking her head. Dr. Tun sighed. "Poor Heidi. Nobody comes to see her. That's why she's acting out."

Carolina nodded as she finished reading the file. "The file says she has a moderate *retraso* [intellectual disability], which means her IQ should be between 35 and 49, but it doesn't say here what her score is. She's been here since March, since right after her mother died."

"And her family hasn't been back," Dr. Tun completed. "We need to get social work out to them, to put some pressure on them. They can't just abandon her here."

"Is she a chronic patient?" I asked.

"No! We don't commit chronic patients anymore," Dr. Tun said firmly.

"The problem is," Carolina explained, summarizing the information she had read in her file, "that we have this young woman. She needs care. Her primary caretaker, her mother, passed away in March. She has siblings, and at first they tried to take her in. First one, then the other. It all fell apart when she accused one of her sibling's sons of raping her. Then they wanted nothing to do with her. She probably made the accusation because of all the changes in her life. She doesn't do well with change. And nobody had the patience to take charge."

"Well she can't stay here," Dr. Tun said again. "They want to abandon her here, but they can't. We will have to put some pressure on them to take responsibility for her."

"They don't know what to do," Carolina continued. "The caretaker she had is leaving, and leaves her in someone else's care. People like her don't do well with change, they are deeply affected by change. They need routine. Meantime, nobody comes to see her, nobody responds when we reach out. Nobody wants to take on the job."

Heidi's story is striking for several reasons. In the first place, Carolina seemed to discount Heidi's claim about being sexually assaulted outright, even though Heidi, as an intellectually disabled woman, was generally more vulnerable to sexual abuse and violence than the general population (DRI 2011, 2015; Hughes et. al. 2012). Instead, Carolina explained Heidi's claims away as a problem of adjustment to change. Meanwhile, while both Dr. Tun and Carolina agreed that Heidi could not be abandoned at Las Lomas, this is, in effect, what her family did. Until the hospital social workers could locate and work with Heidi's family and find a solution, Heidi would have to remain at Las Lomas even though her very presence contradicted the institution's stated goal of deinstitutionalization. Unlike Vannia, who was in her forties with two young children of her own, Heidi was barely out of her teens. Although she was not a minor, she had been brought to the hospital by family members, and the institution saw this family as responsible for her care and future. And while nobody *wanted* Heidi to stay at the hospital when she did not require acute treatment, the inertia of the institution guaranteed that, at the very least, as long as her family succeeded in avoiding phone calls and visits from hospital social workers, Heidi would remain at Las Lomas.

Heidi's story may not be the story of most people who find themselves committed at Las Lomas, but, like that of Doña Isabel, it is not unusual. Despite the institution's official stance, people in Yucatan continue to abandon their unwanted relatives at Las Lomas. The institution becomes a reluctant instrument of structural violence wielded against people like Andrea, Vannia, Doña Isabel, and Heidi. In each case, once the patient is committed, a certain mechanism of action is set into motion whereby each patient must move through the institutional system. When institutional representatives deem a patient unable to take care of herself, it will not release her until some sort of safety net has been established for her. The state strategy of deinstitutionalization is thus undermined by the tactics of people using Las Lomas as a zone of abandonment.

These patients present an ethical challenge for their physicians and the institution. Their needs are not met by psychiatric care, yet they cannot simply be released. As I discuss in the introduction, family played a defining role in who was considered mad in early twentieth-century Mexico (Ríos Molina 2009); likewise, family continues to be extremely important for patient recovery in twenty-first-century Yucatan. While abandonment presents a challenge to the Mexican public mental health care system, most psychiatric patients are not abandoned by their families. For every person like Vannia and Andrea, there are many more people like Brandon's mother (see chapter 2), who found a way to visit Las Lomas every day and assured her son that she was sleeping in the hospital vestibule to make the stay more bearable for him. Psychiatrist Sergio Villaseñor Fajardo's and colleagues' (2003) case study presents an ethnopsychiatric model of inpatient treatment for Mexico that allowed patient family members to stay in the ward with their loved ones; this model was similar to inpatient psychiatric treatment in some resource-poor parts of the world (Watters 2010). In Mexican general (non-psychiatric) hospitals, it is common for family members to stay with the patient for the duration of their hospital stay, and it is relatively rare to find patients in hospitals who are completely alone. Although only a small number among those committed to Las Lomas's wards are abandoned, their stories are similar and numerous enough to suggest that regardless of how the institution sees itself, abandonment continues to occur at Las Lomas. Nearly half of the institution's total number of patient beds are currently occupied by chronic patients.

What is striking about the physical confinement of patients like Andrea, Doña Isabel, Vannia, and Heidi is that they are not committed to Las Lomas because they are experiencing severe psychiatric symptoms. Each of them was left at Las Lomas because no one was willing to care for them outside of the institution: they were abandoned there. Historically, abandonment and local understandings of locura (madness) are intertwined (Sacristán 2005; Ríos Molina 2009). Like today, the presence of a willing outside caretaker was the deciding factor in whether a person was confined. While the women I have described in this chapter may not be suffering from acute psychiatric symptoms, their vulnerability—age, disability, poverty, social isolation—places them into zones of nonbeing (Fanon [1952] 2008), and Las Lomas becomes their Zona del Estar. As the hospital staff tries to figure out what to do with them, all they can do is wait.

In *Vita* (2005), João Biehl first explored the notion of social abandonment, exposing the ways Brazil's entrenched social inequalities and the bureaucratized inefficiency of its medical institutions result in social and biological death. Subsequently, other scholars have explored zones of abandonment and the production of social death (Marrow and Luhrmann 2012; Varley 2016; Leshem 2017). The zone of nonbeing as described in chapter 2 has some interesting parallels with the notion of bare life (Agamben 1995) or Biehl's ex-human—as Grosfoguel has frequently pointed out, a decolonial perspective embraces epistemic plurality and accepts that no epistemology has a monopoly on an objective "truth." Agamben's bare life and Biehl's ex-human speak to the way that social abandonment leads to social—and, eventually, biological—death. However, nonbeing is not equivalent to social death, and Las Lomas is not a zone of social death, or even, arguably, a zone of social abandonment. The patients described here are in a zone of nonbeing because they have been stripped of what makes them full persons in any modern society—self-determination—but they are still very much socially alive. The institution must house, feed, and medicate them. It cannot simply release them into the street to fend for themselves. Every patient I have described (with the exception of Andrea, who caused consternation nonetheless even if nothing was done to investigate) was a source of concern for the institution's representatives.

Las Lomas staff understood that Heidi, Vannia, and Doña Isabel should not stay permanently at the hospital, but they could not simply be released without somewhere to go and someone to care for them. Structural constraints put the institution in a bind: while the underlying ethos of the institution aligns with international law that states that psychiatric patients and other people with physical and intellectual disabilities should reside in their communities and be provided with resources and treatment that allow them to live independently and thrive outside of an institutional setting, these resources simply do not exist (DRI 2011). When a patient is involuntarily committed, she becomes the legal responsibility of the institution. Without a clear plan for her care, the institution cannot release her. Efforts are made to either locate family to hold responsible or place her somewhere outside the institution. Las Lomas, like the psychiatric hospital described by Biehl in Vita, is a stopping point, a holding place of sorts, not a destination. Zona del Estar, characterized by a temporality of the present (and temporalized presence), presents a useful framework for thinking about madness and confinement in the colonial matrix of power.

In his exploration of the psychiatric hospital that brought so much harm to Catarina, Biehl notes that psychiatric institutions can transform people into "pharmaceutical beings" (2005, 199). At Las Lomas, biomedically minded psychiatrists and residents are trained to rely primarily on pharmaceuticals, particularly when caring for patients who are committed. This is not unusual but is in fact consistent with biomedical psychiatry in the Global North, which increasingly focuses on pharmaceutical treatment in preference to psychodynamic approaches to treatment or psychotherapy (Luhrmann 2000). Dr. Tun was an anomaly because even though she medicated every patient under her care, she did not medicate them *enough*, at least in the opinion of her nursing staff. It was Andrea's *lack* of medication that perplexed Dr. Tun and made Andrea so anomalous. Thus, while Las Lomas may have been a stopping point for each of the patients described in this chapter (all of whom had been abandoned in some way), this stopping point carries long-term consequences, which reflected the inertia of the bureaucracy within the institution and beyond, as the patients' stays became prolonged. In each case, these patients were involuntarily confined and had been deserted by their families and dismissed by their medical providers.

As I discuss in chapter 4, the prevention of institutionalization is a primary purpose of Las Lomas: the institution's goal is the creation and rehabilitation of neoliberal, rational, self-governing subjects capable of functioning in society. The idea of madness has been abandoned in favor of notions of mental health and mental illness. The term *usuario* (user) has replaced *paciente* (patient), which itself replaced *loco* (lunatic). Yet, the continual use of Las Lomas as a zone of abandonment by people who are outside the institution undermines its purpose. By the same token, the inaccessibility of the experiences of patients, local authorities, and family members prior to and following hospitalization presents a serious methodological challenge. I simply cannot know, based on the data available, how the decision to abandon is made. We only know what the file says, and the file cannot always be trusted. However, once the patient is initially confined, the status of the patient as a person changes from that of a rights-holding citizen to that of a legal ward and body that must be managed.

MAKING THE MATRIX

Writing this chapter was remarkably difficult because it took me some time to realize why I kept putting three very different phenomena—the role of personal relationships and party politics in the institution, the practice of illegally doubling up on public insurance, and the obstinacy of the asylum model and prevalence of abandonment in the neoliberal hospital—in a single chapter. After many frustrated drafts and attempts to pull the three apart, I realized why I kept putting them together: the colonial matrix of power can only be understood as an enormous web of social processes and relationships. Each of these instances illustrates how the colonial matrix of power is constituted into being. Each instance contains within it multiple interactions taking place among individual actors, medical systems, and the state itself. The events I have described showcase the capillary functioning of coloniality as people act within the scope of their agency to resist and propagate social structure, often simultaneously.

Quijano might not like to have his framework of the colonial matrix of power compared to the Wachowskis' 1999 science fiction film, *The Matrix*, which depicted a society in which self-aware computers have enslaved humanity and maintain control by keeping the human population in stasis, wherein people experience a computer-generated virtual reality world for the entirety of their existence. This film has been thoroughly analyzed in other scholarly literature (Diocaretz and Herbrechter 2006; Stucky 2005), though perhaps not from this perspective. The film does lend itself to this small comparison. In *The Matrix*, humanity is docile because it is unaware that its social existence has been constructed by an exploitative power. Humans live out their lives within the constraints of the reality imposed upon them for the benefit of others. Similarly, in the colonial matrix of power, human beings remain largely unaware of the ways in which their actions and reactions—their tactics in the face of state strategy—further constitute and re-entrench the world as they know it.

Nevertheless, the real world is not *The Matrix*. While the stories of patients from Las Lomas show the ways in which the colonial matrix of power is constituted through a series of small-scale actions and social processes, they also demonstrate the complexity of everyday life. Fortunes change, careers are made and lost, and what was once taken for granted disappears or changes form. Through it all, life goes on, and so does its practice.

4 · MODERNITY

Problem and Promise of Mexican Psychiatry

Nos pusieron a lado del basurero municipal. Por supuesto que entendimos el mensaje.

They put us next to the city dump. Of course, we got the message.
—Dr. Juan Vasquez, Las Lomas

Located at the end of a street, next to a beautiful city park, Las Lomas is a 160-bed psychiatric facility in the Merida metropolitan area. In 2011, the facility provided inpatient and outpatient services to 69,000 people. The hospital had four inpatient wards (intensive care, chronic care, and separate long-term men's and women's wards). It also had a psychiatric emergency room where patients are assessed prior to admission, an outpatient care program that includes individual psychiatric monitoring and individual and group therapy, and it provided pediatric psychiatry services. A sprawling campus dotted with a series of squat, single-story structures, Las Lomas opened its doors in 1971, when it was moved from what is today Centro Estatal de Bellas Artes, the state-sponsored School of Fine Arts. The old building is located across the street from the city zoo, which opened in 1910 in celebration of the nation's centennial. Juan and his old friend and mentor, Dr. Manuel Treviño, reminisced one day as I asked them about Las Lomas's history.[1] Both physicians were there when it first opened, and Dr. Treviño had previously worked at the old psychiatric hospital. Both Dr. Vásquez and Dr. Treviño were born and raised in Yucatan, and Dr. Treviño was close to seventy when I first met him in 2008.

"It was part of *Domingo Familiar* [Family Sunday], you know," Dr. Treviño chuckled as he remembered the old institution. "Parents would take their children to the *Centenario* [zoo][2] to see the lions, and then cross the street to look on at *los loquitos* [the lunatics]. This was in the days where all we had was insulin treatment. Oh, what terrible times those were." He leaned back in his chair, his large belly making the buttons on his guayabera (shirt) stretch, and looked at me with twinkling blue eyes. "Pharmaceuticals have transformed the quality of life for our patients, especially the schizophrenics. You should know that. I remember what it was like before we had them." Dr. Treviño's description is very similar to that of other Mexican psychiatrists who practiced at psychiatric hospitals prior to the late 1950s, when the first pharmaceuticals were introduced (Calderón Narváez 1996a, 1996b, 2002; Fernández del Castillo 1966; Sacristán 2005).

Juan never said much about the old hospital, where he volunteered as a medical student, save to point out for me the last person to be lobotomized there, a man who continues to reside at Las Lomas but who is allowed to come and go, selling pastries on the streets to generate an income. In a recent conversation, he told me the old Hospital Ayala was "horror-inducing." About ten of Las Lomas's oldest permanently committed patients were originally committed to the old Hospital Ayala and moved to Las Lomas, where it is expected they will live out the rest of their lives. Juan also pointed out something about the *new* hospital, the location where Las Lomas was built. Today, a large city park is located right next to Las Lomas. Runners, children, and students from a nearby high school like to frequent it, as do the owners of food carts selling churros, hot dogs, and *marquesitas*, a local delicacy. But in 1978, where the park is today was the city dump. For Juan, the symbolism was impossible to miss. "The hospital was supposed to be on the cutting edge. It was going to bring us into modernity. A true twentieth century facility. But they put us next to the city dump. Of course, we got the message, we were psychoanalysts!!" The hospital, decrepit and nearly crumbling apart when I first entered it thirty years later, was lauded as a revolution in mental health care: the medicalization of the facility was a decided move away from "ineffective" psychoanalytic approaches and toward the reconceptualization of mental illness as biological suffering that emerged at the same time as the anti-psychiatry movement, which rejected the very idea of mental illness as anything other than a variation of normal. As pharmaceuticals revolutionized the treatment of severe mental illness, the anti-psychiatry movement challenged the use of invasive interventions such as electroconvulsive therapy, insulin shock therapy, malaria therapy, and psychosurgical interventions like lobotomy. These fell by the wayside with the emergence of pharmaceuticals.

Yucatecan psychiatry entered the twentieth century, but—if Juan, who directed the institution for eighteen years, from 1982 to 2000, is to be believed—this "entrance" was disingenuous. By building the hospital next to the city dump, the state government symbolically identified the mentally ill patients using its services, along with the priorities of the new institution, with trash. Likewise, the new hospital's employees would be among the lowest-paid in the country, and the psychiatric profession would continue to suffer a reputation for being "unscientific," "not real doctors," or simply *loqueros* (doctors of the mad).

At the same time, Las Lomas's history is embedded in the broader history of medicine in Mexico. The pharmaceutical revolution transformed the practice of psychiatry itself. The emergence of modern medical discourses emphasizing recovery, self-sufficiency, and social integration further transformed Las Lomas from an asylum to a psychiatric hospital. Juan oversaw the further organization of the hospital into its current form. It was Juan who introduced the emergency room and the acute ward, both of which use names borrowed from nonpsychiatric hospitals: *urgencias* (emergency) and *cuidados intensivos* (intensive care). As he confirmed when I asked him, this was not coincidental: the goal was to make Las Lomas resemble a "real" hospital as much as possible, alongside making hospital stays shorter and committing patients as infrequently as possible.

One day in July 2012, I was sitting in on Juan's appointments. His office was located in the administrative wing of the hospital. It was a comfortable space with a window (a curtain drawn over it for privacy) looking out into the hallway and air conditioning that Juan had paid to install.

His first appointment, Dora, walked in. She was a thin woman in her late fifties.

"This is Betty," Juan explained. "She is an anthropologist. She is with me today to observe my *consulta*. Is that okay?"

She smiled at me and nodded, but did not say anything.

"So, how's it going, Dora? How is everything?"

Dora's jaw quivered, her eyes filled with tears. She spent the next twenty minutes explaining her conflicts with family members, her struggle to get up each morning, her feelings of loneliness. Juan listened, asked questions, and—in a fashion very unlike that of psychiatry as it is practiced in the United States—offered occasional advice. At the end of the *consulta*, Juan wrote her a new prescription for her medications, explaining he was not going to change them today, and handed them to her. Dora looked at the pieces of paper in her hand and looked up, a glimmer of hope in her eyes.

"Can't I stay here today, doctor?"

Juan let out an exaggerated chuckle. "Stay? You don't want to stay here! Listen, it's Friday. Get your medication, take a few days, come back on Monday, okay? If you still want to stay we can discuss it then. How does that sound?"

She nodded in agreement, "*Está bien. El lunes, pues* [Okay, then, Monday]."

After she left Juan turned to me.

"You see? Some of them, after that initial stay here, they like it. They want to come back, to stay here because it gets them away from what they are dealing with at home. It's the idea of the asylum, persistent as it is. They seek refuge. But we're not supposed to be about that, no. We are supposed to keep them out as much as we can. The biomedical model of psychiatry at work, you see? Focus on the biochemistry, treat the brain. But the patients, they still see the hospital as an asylum."

I nodded as he spoke, scribbling notes and thinking. At this point, in the summer of 2012, Juan and I had known each other for four years. We had had this conversation many times. At first glance, Juan's discourse can be read simply as a reflection on two different ways of understanding mental illness: the premodern asylum and the modern hospital (Foucault 1988b). Juan's interest in keeping Dora out of Las Lomas may appear to be quite congruent with the genealogy of the "psy" sciences as described by Nikolas Rose (1996). Rose presents a linear narrative by which scientific knowledge of the mind and mental illness—the "psy" sciences—emerge from an institutional need to anticipate and control human behavior. Rose follows Foucault's argument that psychiatry essentially functions as a mechanism of social regulation and control, at the same time he notes that this mechanism is displaced from social institutions into individual subjective bodies: the responsibility for social regulation and control is expected to be owned by a (modern) individual, self-actualizing subject. Foucault once referred to psychiatric patients and other subaltern peoples as the possessors of "subjugated knowledges" (1972), and the anti-psychiatric movement challenged the notion of mental illness itself. Under this perspective, the diversity of human experience and other ways of knowing and experiencing the world are subjugated to the rational expectations of post-Enlightenment modernity. In this sense, one can observe the "psy" sciences as part of the process of colonization, the extension of the colonizing force into the mind—articulated by Fanon in *The Wretched of the Earth*. Under this analysis, Juan's perspective reflects a psychiatric sensitivity congruent with other modern logics of the Global North. There is more to this encounter, however, than meets the eye.

Rather than merely replicate the trajectory of the "psy" sciences in the Global North, Mexican psychiatry has its own historical particularities.[3] Frankfurt School psychoanalyst Erich Fromm (1900–1980), a founder of the psychoanalytic program at the national Universidad Nacional Autónoma de México (UNAM) and known as the father of socialist humanism, played an important role in the formation of Mexican psychiatry through his involvement with Mexico's Manicomio General de la Castañeda in the 1950s (Calderón Narváez 1996b). Fromm's psychoanalysis was heavily influenced by Marx as well as Freud. While Frommian psychology is still reliant on Freudian notions of the unconscious, it breaks away from some of the binary reasoning in Freudian thought (such as the conceived oppositions of desire and repression) toward the notion of "orientations," based on the ways in which human beings engage with one another in the world in relationships that can be nonproductive (receptive, exploitative, hoarding, marketing) or "productive," the potential of all human beings to love and affirm each other (Fromm 1990). To return to Dora's story, while Juan is treating Dora pharmacologically, his interest in keeping her out of the institution is connected to his Frommian orientation, which is to help Dora develop a productive (defined as healthy, nonexploitative, and affirming) relationship with her family and others around her.

Fromm's socialist psychology essentially married sociology and psychology, an approach that found ready acceptance in Mexico, where he spent the final twenty-five years of his career (de Rodrigo 2015; Funk 2003). At Las Lomas, psychoanalytically oriented psychiatrists like Drs. Vasquez, Treviño, and Tun all characterize themselves as heavily influenced by Frommian thought, as do many practicing psychologists. This orientation frames the way in which Dr. Vasquez and his colleagues understand the role of self in society. The biomedicalization of psychiatry has occurred alongside the neoliberalization of Mexican society—fewer and fewer psychiatrists are interested in pursuing psychoanalytic frameworks, focusing almost exclusively on psychopharmacology. It is perhaps ironic that, toward the end of his life, Fromm referred to then-nascent neoliberalism as a "pathology of normality"—the displacement of productive human relationships in favor of self-serving exploitation (de Rodrigo 2015). The biomedicalization of psychiatry and its underlying therapeutic ethos (Illouz 2008) are inherently characteristic of modern medicine. At heart is an assumption of what is desired of the psychiatric patient and what "recovery" actually means. In Mexico, this is not merely the emergence and dominance of a European subjectivity and individual self-care, but rather the convergence of these logics with older yet salient medical and state paternalism, and locally defined understandings of health, illness, and the self.

While international organizations like Disability Rights International have issued reports focused on the fates of the many people trapped without recourse in Mexican psychiatric institutions (DRI 2011, 2015; MDRI 2000), Dora was not the first nor the only patient I ever encountered who seemed to *want* to be inside Las Lomas. Lina, whose story I return to at several points in this book, also wanted to be committed, albeit probably for different reasons. While Las Lomas is guided by an ethos typical of many neoliberal institutions in the Global North—the transformation of the mad into rational, self-actualizing neoliberal subjects (Foucault 1988a, 1988b; Rose 1996), the people who walk through its doors and wards do not always behave or become what the institution desires for them. The reasons for this are many, as I explore throughout this book. The incomplete mission of the Mexican psychiatric hospital is intimately connected to the colonial experience of modernity in contemporary Mexico. Culture, political economy, competing interests, politics, and epistemologies encounter each other and produce an organized chaos that can only be described as a collection of human beings trying to keep their humanity in inhumane conditions, a messy system of loose ends and unresolved tensions carried forward by its inertia as it endlessly creates and recreates some version of Quijano's colonial matrix of power. This chapter is a guided tour of Las Lomas, its history within the greater history of Mexican psychiatry, guiding ethos, and inhabitants (providers and patients alike). It provides a road map, so to speak, to better understand the psychiatric encounters described in the rest of this book.

Dr. Juan Vasquez, my main interlocutor at Las Lomas, is a jovial, charismatic man. In his sixties at the time of this writing, he rides a Harley Davidson motorcycle from his home just north of Merida to Las Lomas, which is located in what used to be a peripheral community on the other side of the city. Juan is the reason I began conducting research at Las Lomas. A psychiatrist who holds a master's degree in anthropology, he invited me to study La Esperanza, Las Lomas's suicide prevention program, in 2008. My work with Esperanza included participant observation at Las Lomas, sitting in on various small and large group therapy and support sessions as well as participating in a weekly reading group where Juan and his team—a group of psychologists, residents, and community volunteers—read the works of Mexican and other Latin American ethnopsychiatrists, classic works like Durkheim's *Le Suicide*, and any literature that combined suicide and sociological or anthropological approaches. The work in 2008 was difficult and rewarding beyond measure. I left Yucatan in December 2008 feeling like I had more work to do. After I completed my PhD studies, I started to think about this unfinished work. Juan invited me to return to Las Lomas and continue my work, an invitation I gladly accepted.

There were stark differences in both my research interest and my ethnographic approach on my second trip to Las Lomas. Unlike my first visit, I was there to study health care delivery, not suicide prevention. Thus, unlike my previous visit, where my interactions in Las Lomas had been limited to its almost entirely volunteer-operated suicide prevention program, La Esperanza, this time I was given permission to enter the wards themselves. I soon divided my time between the acute care ward, the emergency room, and outpatient services. I found myself sitting in on clinical case discussions, occasionally being asked to provide input from an anthropological perspective. Over the years, I came to know and understand the psychiatric facility quite well.

ON THE INSIDE: A GUIDED TOUR

All newly admitted patients spend at least two days in the ICU ward before they are transferred to the "gardens" or long-term ward. To reach it, one must check in with the security guard sitting at the back entrance of the main building and supply him with one's identification. Then, one has to walk down a walkway behind the main building, pass the hospital cafeteria and classrooms, and head toward the back of the property. The ward is a white, one-story, cement-block structure with two small wings, one on either side. Its entrance is closed by two black metal doors that can be opened only with a key and have no outside handle. During the day, the doors remain open. The doors open into a wide, long hallway connecting the two wings. Directly across from the ward entrance is another door, leading to a courtyard. On the right side of the courtyard is an entrance marked "residency," and at the end of the courtyard are the staff bathrooms. Immediately to the right, a door marked *enfermería* (nursing) leads to the nurses' office. Next to this door is a desk that is occasionally used by the ward's social worker, and behind it, around the corner, is the long room that houses the hospital's ECT machine. Along the wall immediately next to this room are Dr. Pacheco's and Dr. Tun's offices, and across the hall—in a room with a wall made of decorative masonry blocks allowing visual observation—is the isolation room, containing one bed and its own bathroom.

At the other end of the hall are two offices. One was used for storage, the other belonged to Dr. Castro, the attending psychiatrist to the men in the ICU. Dr. Castro's office is spare: a desk, two metal and plastic chairs, and nothing else. It did not appear as if Dr. Castro kept any personal property inside his office. The most distinctive feature was a machine in the wall that looked like it belonged on a submarine. Dr. Castro explained that it was an old instrument sanitizer. It had not been used in many years. I wondered at the time if patients, scared and confused and possibly delusional, might not think it was some kind of torture device.

To the right of Dr. Castro's office is the men's dormitory, and to the left is the women's. The dormitories are long rooms, with metal hospital beds with black rubber mattresses. At the end of the room, showerheads are visible; a low wall just before them discreetly hides the toilets. Outside the dormitories, in the hallway, is the nurses' station, a table where nurses sit between tasks during their shifts. Both dormitories are clearly visible from the nurses' station through windows lined with decorative masonry blocks.

The building is not air conditioned. A cross-breeze is created by opening the building's doors and windows, but the absence of mosquito netting and the preponderance of places for stagnant water to accumulate means that once the rainy season starts, the building is overrun with mosquitoes, and the risk of patients contracting mosquito-borne diseases such as dengue fever and chikungunya is high. The doctors and staff cope by bringing in fly swatters—a particularly effective one is shaped like a racket and contains an electrical charge. When mosquitoes come into contact with the racket's metal strings, they die, releasing the distinctive smell of burnt blood if they have recently feasted. The patients, who are allowed no personal property, have no such recourse, and simply have to endure them.

Dr. Tun's office has one unique feature: an air conditioner. Dr. Tun bought the unit herself and had it installed in her office, which contains a desk, a medical scale, and an examination table. It also contains some personal items: a glass vase with some artificial flowers and a red valentine heart sit in the shelves on the wall. There are hooks on the wall, with a wire hanger on which Dr. Tun hangs her white doctor's coat at the end of each day. Compared to Dr. Pacheco and Dr. Castro's offices, Dr. Tun's office gives the impression that she has made some effort to make the space her own.

Dr. Pacheco's office has a desk, two chairs, and a cot against the back wall. The room also holds a medical scale and an empty storage cabinet. A closet faces the window. Unlike Dr. Tun's office, Dr. Pacheco's office does not have an air conditioner. He prefers to open the windows, without mosquito netting, for natural light. His window overlooks the yard of the long-term ward. When he brings patients in for their daily consultation, it is not unusual for other patients to stand outside the open windows, leaning their arms against the glass. Dr. Pacheco knows them well.

"Come back later, Teófilo," he'll say, not unkindly, to a young, developmentally challenged man peeking in, "I'll call you when I'm ready." And Teófilo will wander away.

Through the window, I can see the building housing the men's long-term ward. Two state police officers stand outside the door, chatting amiably with each other and with the doctors and nurses passing by. Sometimes, I see them sitting at a table with a checkers board painted on its surface. They are there as custodians of patients who were committed after an arrest; in local parlance, these patients are *en calidad de detenido*, detained due to criminal charges.

Also, unlike Dr. Tun's office, Dr. Pacheco's office has two doors, each facing a ward. This is because Dr. Pacheco, as the only IMSS psychiatrist, cares for his patients from the moment they are committed through the moment they are released. Most patients committed to the ICU are not released back home but are transferred into the long-term ward, and so Dr. Pacheco needs access to his patients in both wards to provide continuity of care. Of the three attending physicians, Dr. Pacheco was able to develop the most meaningful relationships with his patients because of this.

Patients walking into the emergency room for the first time will enter the hospital through the main entrance, pass the vendors who set up tables in the hospital vestibule to sell food, religious texts, or the latest Herbalife products, and be directed to the last door on the left, at the end of the corridor to the right of the main entrance. If the door is closed, the patients must knock on it, and a psychiatry resident wearing a white doctor's coat will open it. This door leads to a room with yet another door on the opposite wall. The room contains a desk, a chair, and an examination table. Beyond this door is another room—this one air-conditioned—with yet another desk, a few more chairs, and another examination table. To the right of the desk facing this door is another door that opens to a room with two hospital beds, a crash cart containing a defibrillator (medical equipment used in cardiac arrest), and a medication cabinet. Then, beyond that is an ominous-looking gated doorway with vertical bars. This is the room where patients who are committed must leave their families and loved ones behind. Here, too, patients must change from their own clothing into the hospital uniform; if they refuse to change themselves, the nurses will do it for them. In my time at Las Lomas, I only saw an involuntary commitment happen once—it seemed that many of these commitments, particularly the ones where patients were subjected to the forcible changing of their clothes, tended to happen overnight. The overnight shift is usually attended by a contract psychiatrist supervising a resident.

In his role as emergency room attending physician, Dr. Patrón was a primary gatekeeper of the institution: his job was to assess patients who came into the emergency room, and then recommend whether a patient went home or was admitted for inpatient treatment. Theoretically, patients who were going through a psychiatric emergency—people experiencing a psychotic break, suicidal ideation, a manic or depressive state—are assessed, and the attending psychiatrist then decides whether to admit them or prescribe a short-term medication regimen and refer them to outpatient treatment. Some patients were referred to Las Lomas from other hospitals, particularly following suicide attempts. Others were brought by ambulance from their home communities. Many, having exhausted options locally available to them—local clinics and traditional medical practitioners such as yerbateros and hmeeno'ob—will walk in to the Las Lomas emergency room as a first step toward accessing regular outpatient treatment. As I note in the introduction and elsewhere (Reyes-Foster 2013a, 2016a), local etiologies generally link mental illness to spiritual and social malaise but are on the whole compatible with biomedical models of care. Thus, a patient struggling with psychiatric symptoms will likely rely on a combination of pharmaceutical treatment, traditional medicine, and catholic prayer without seeing any contradiction between the multiple etiologies informing each approach. Generally speaking, by the time a patient arrives at the psychiatric emergency room in Las Lomas, all of these approaches will have been exhausted with little relief.

In most cases, Dr. Patrón would prescribe medication—depending on the symptoms, mood stabilizers, antipsychotics, benzodiazepenes, antidepressants—and send patients on their way with instructions to return for follow-up with him, usually within a week. Explaining that he believed most patients should be treated at home and avoid possible trauma of institutionalization, he avoided admitting patients as much as possible. Dr. Patrón, like many of his colleagues inside and outside the institution, saw Las Lomas as a resource of last resort.

There was only one instance where I directly witnessed Dr. Patrón offer to admit a patient. A young couple, Manuel and Carmen, came to consult Dr. Patrón in the emergency room. As they came in to the room, a nurse followed them, holding a patient file. Manuel, who suffered from schizophrenia, had already been previously committed to Las Lomas. He and Carmen sat across from Dr. Patrón. Carmen explained he had stopped taking his medication and was hearing voices again.

"He's accusing me of cheating on him," she explained. "He won't be persuaded otherwise. He's hearing things that aren't there. He denies it, but I've caught him arguing with himself."

Her husband sat next to hear, his arms crossed, glowering at her.

"Has he been violent toward you?" Dr. Patrón asked.

The two exchanged a meaningful glance, but when she turned back to us she shook her head no.

Dr. Patrón tried to get Manuel to answer some orientation questions—What is your name? Where are we? What is today's date—before asking about his symptoms. The more Dr. Patrón asked about voices, the more agitated Manuel became. Finally, Manuel admitted that the voices he was hearing were telling him that his wife was having an affair, and this was making him angry.

"Have you been violent towards your wife?" Dr. Patrón asked again.

"Only because she's cheating on me!" Manuel finally burst out, "if she weren't cheating on me I wouldn't have to beat her up!"

This seemed to confirm Dr. Patrón's suspicions. He turned toward Carmen. "At this point it is evident that your husband is experiencing psychosis and that he could be violent towards you. I am offering to admit him right now. We can medicate him and get his symptoms under control. The decision is yours."

Carmen looked timidly at Manuel. "Do you want to stay, Manuel?"

Manuel replied with a glower. She turned toward us. "He doesn't want to stay."

"That may be," Dr. Patrón replied, "but this is not his decision. It is yours. I am offering to admit him. He can stay right now."

Manuel's glower deepened. Carmen looked back at him. Something crossed between them, and she looked back at Dr. Patrón. "No. Not today."

Dr. Patrón wrote a prescription for an antipsychotic and admonished Manuel to take it and come back in seven days for follow-up. After they left, we remarked about the palpable tension we had felt in the room. Dr. Patrón shook his head. "I have no doubt she's going home to another beating," he said. "She should have let me admit him."

We did not see them again.

Manuel and Carmen's case highlights several important facts to keep in mind when considering how patients are admitted to Las Lomas: in the first instance, admission is usually offered only when the attending physician has a concern about the safety of the patient or those around him. Second, this admission can be declined by the patient's legal representative—in Manuel and Carmen's case, once Dr. Patrón determined that Manuel was ill enough to warrant admitting, Carmen became his legal guardian. She had the power to consent to his admission to Las Lomas, and—had he been admitted—the power to sign him out or consent to invasive treatment such as electroconvulsive therapy (ECT). She would have been considered legally responsible for his well-being.

PSYCHIATRIC INSTITUTIONS IN MEXICO

There are thirty-one psychiatric hospitals in operation in Mexico today, holding approximately 7,000 patients (DRI 2011). A Disability Rights International report published in 2000 found massive human rights violations in Mexico's mental health system. Follow-up investigations ten and fifteen years later found "almost no change" (DRI 2011, viii) in violations despite federal government commitments to addressing rampant abuses in its psychiatric hospitals. A 2011 report found widespread abuse of physical restraints, psychosurgery (including lobotomy), and inhumane, degrading living conditions. The conditions at Las Lomas as I observed them seemed better than those described in these reports, although I witnessed a fair number of people who were overmedicated, physically restrained, and locked up in closed wards. I saw what—at least to an outsider—appeared to be an overly easy reliance on ECT. Yet, at the same time, the people I worked with over years of research were not intentionally malicious or abusive. They recognized and bemoaned many of the problems identified in the DRI reports. They struggled to provide quality care in an underfunded institution where medication shortages were frequent, the facilities were falling apart, and patients had few resources on the outside to prevent relapse and rehospitalization.

To understand how Las Lomas functions, it is important to understand how people in Mexico access health care, especially mental health care services, today. Health care delivery in Mexico can be a complicated affair. The federal government operates four state-sponsored, socialized health care schemes, each with its own hospitals, clinics, and infrastructure. These are the once-beloved *Instituto Mexicano del Seguro Social* (IMSS), created for private-sector employees and partially funded by employers; the *Instituto de Seguridad Social de Trabajadores del Estado* (ISSSTE), created for federal government employees; and *Seguro Popular*, for those who are self-, under-, or unemployed or otherwise do not have access to IMSS or ISSSTE.[4] At the state level, Instituto de Seguridad Social para los Trabajadores del Estado de Yucatan (ISSSTEY) funds state employee health care in regular IMSS facilities. Other large employers, such as the Universidad Autónoma de Yucatan (UADY), have their own health care systems using a combination of their own infrastructure and contracting with private providers and facilities.

Lauded as a breakthrough when it was launched in 2004, Seguro Popular created access to health care for 55 million uninsured Mexicans. Under the auspices of the *Secretaría de Salud* (the Mexican public health secretariat), the program absorbed a decrepit and underfunded system of facilities that had up until then been providing free but mostly inadequate care. Alongside the acquisition of this existing infrastructure, the new program set about building gleaming new facilities throughout the country to provide highly specialized care. Despite the conspicuous construction of these new facilities, Seguro Popular has received mixed reviews (Homedes and Ugalde 2009; Támez González and Valle Arcos 2005). Because it is in line with neoliberal approaches to health reforms that displace responsibility for population health on to individual consumers of health, critics have accused proponents of Seguro Popular of attempting to undermine the IMSS system, which is widely seen as diametrically opposed in its ethos and mission (Hayden 2007).

By the same token, alternative medical systems exist. Most middle- and upper-class Mexicans, even when they have access to IMSS or ISSSTE, prefer to use private health care providers when possible. This has created a thriving private health insurance market, in which Mexicans who can afford it will purchase coverage for major medical expenses such as hospitalizations and catastrophic illness. The private sector remains relatively affordable, which leads many Mexicans, even some who may be considered poor, to opt to pay for private care from time to time (see, for instance, Chelito's story in chapter 2). At the same time, low-cost pharmacies—spearheaded by Farmacias Similares, a pharmaceutical laboratory specializing in generics—also provide free or extremely low-cost medical consultations. However, extremely low-cost pharmacies like Similares do not sell highly controlled medications such as the benzodiazepines—clonazepam and alprazolam—two of the most prescribed medications at Las Lomas. These medications are usually obtained through the public medical systems or private pharmacies.

As I discussed in chapter 1, in addition to mental health care services provided by the state and an array of private medical and psychological practitioners, people who reside in Yucatan's rural communities or even in its poorer urban neighborhoods have access to traditional medical practitioners. These are hmeeno'ob, hueseros, and yerbateros who treat a variety of ailments using a humoral etiology, whereby symptoms may be caused by *nervios* (nerves), *susto* (shock or fear), *ojo* (evil eye), *malos vientos* (bad winds), wandering organs, humoral imbalance between hot and cold, or witchcraft. Each of these specialists treat symptoms differently—where hueseros are essentially bone-setters who also provide treatment using massage, yerbateros are herbal specialists. Hmeen'o'ob, on the other hand, are shamanic priests. Although they have extensive knowledge of the use of plants for medical treatment, much of the work they do involves the invocation of spirits and the performance of rituals that heal individuals, entire communities, or even places. Their role as healers is intertwined with their role as spiritual interlocutors. Although some of these practitioners are nominally integrated into the Mexican medical system under the auspices of *interculturalidad* (see the next section in this chapter), most are not.

As I (Reyes-Foster 2013, 2016) and others (Duncan 2017) have pointed out, most patients do not perceive these medical systems as being exclusive of one another. By the time they arrive at Las Lomas, for instance, many patients who come from outside the city of Merida have already exhausted other options, including psychological services locally available to them and traditional medicine. In fact, many people who experience psychological distress never make it to Merida or Las Lomas simply because they are able to recover using a combination of locally available services, as I describe, for instance, in the case of Xulab (Reyes-Foster 2013a, 2016), where villagers were able to address their anxieties following the suicides of two young girls by using a combination of psychological treatment, traditional medicine, and prayer.

So where in this huge and complex system does Las Lomas fit in? Officially, Las Lomas is owned and operated by Salubridad and should, theoretically, be funded primarily through Seguro Popular. However, though the programs are supposed to operate independently of each other, Las Lomas's inpatient facilities are also contracted out to IMSS and ISSSTE, and IMSS and ISSSTE psychiatrists use a different office than other Las Lomas psychiatrists. Dr. Pacheco, the IMSS psychiatrist, uses his office in the mornings, and the same office is used by Dr. Maduro, the ISSSTE psychiatrist, in the afternoons. IMSS and ISSSTE patients wear blue hospital gowns whereas other patients wear green hospital gowns. Although these IMSS and ISSSTE patients sleep in the same dormitories and are treated by the same nurses, their treatment is overseen by a non–Las Lomas psychiatrist. They are not assessed or treated by residents. More importantly, as already noted, their treatment is overseen by the same psychiatrist from the time they are admitted (unless they are admitted with unknown insurance status) to the time they are released, allowing for more complete continuity of care.

A frequent point of confusion, however, comes when patients are initially admitted. Patients are often admitted with unknown insurance status. Even when insurance status is known, family members must go through a formal approval process and file several forms of paperwork, requiring them to travel between Las Lomas and their own locally assigned IMSS or ISSSTE treatment facility to have the patients' care transferred to the IMSS or ISSSTE psychiatrist. This long and cumbersome process interrupts continuity of care, as patients will be treated by the Las Lomas attending psychiatrist—in this case, Dr. Tun or Dr. Pacheco—until the process is completed. After this, they will not see them again. In the acute ward, where trust and connection are crucial to successful treatment, these interruptions and vacillations are a serious challenge to effective treatment.

The reason patients are often admitted with unknown insurance status is that only patients who are deemed to be in an extreme crisis are admitted at Las Lomas. In my conversations with psychiatrists working at Las Lomas and in other local hospitals, I found that psychiatrists avoid referring patients to Las Lomas whenever possible. In my own observations of the psychiatric emergency room, usually a first point of contact between patients and Las Lomas, Dr. Patrón, the ER psychiatrist, often examined patients, prescribed medications, and asked them to return for a follow-up. Psychiatrists working in local hospitals usually opted to refer their patients to outpatient care rather than send them to Las Lomas, in part because of Las Lomas's terrible reputation. People outside the hospital, even other psychiatrists, describe Las Lomas as a broken institution full of misfits, staffed by "doctors who aren't even psychiatrists," as one psychiatrist who did not work at Las Lomas stated. This refers to a widespread belief that hospital psychiatrists are medical doctors who did not complete a psychiatry residency program but came to specialize in psychiatry by focusing their medical practice on this particular patient population (a common practice for many medical specializations in the past).[5]

Many patients who are admitted come from rural zones located long distances from the hospital. They face significant obstacles in accessing care: first, depending on the remoteness of their residence, they may not have regular access to a psychiatrist or another mental health care provider; second, even with access to medical care, medication shortages are common in Mexico's public hospitals and clinics; finally, using the services of a mental health care professional or a psychiatrist is not a common cultural practice, though this care is becoming increasingly available in larger towns such as Valladolid, Ticul, and Tizimín. By the time they are committed, most patients have already made use of local traditional medicine options available to them. For many, these healers, used alongside local health care providers, are enough. However, when locally available care fails and patients experience a crisis, they may find themselves transported to Las Lomas. In the end, most patients committed to Las Lomas fall under Seguro Popular or are uninsured. Dr. Pacheco and Dr. Maduro's patient rosters are usually quite small, with numbers fewer than ten and sometimes as low as two or three at any one time.

NEOLIBERAL SUBJECTIVITY AND *INTERCULTURALIDAD*

The twenty-first century has become characterized by the expansion and pervasiveness of neoliberal economic policy. A reiteration of late nineteenth-century laissez-faire economics, neoliberalism is characterized by an emphasis on free, unregulated markets and consumer-driven economies. However, as a number of scholars (Biehl, Good, and Kleinman 2007; Lakoff 2005; Rose 1996) have pointed out, neoliberalism represents much more than a pervasive economic system; it encapsulates an ideology about governance, citizenship, and ultimately subjectivity. Rose is specifically interested in the emergence of *neoliberal subjectivity*, a subjectivity characterized by governmentality: the transfer of governance from an outside entity (the state) to the subject. Under this perspective, neoliberal subjects are rational, self-interested, and self-actualizing. This premise—that modern subjects will act in their own self-interest—characterizes the approaches of development programs such as microlending in developing countries around the world. As Appadurai (1996) described more than twenty years ago, contemporary societies are characterized by "flows" and "-scapes," which are largely facilitated by an economic system that recognizes fewer and fewer boundaries. People, money, and technologies flow over borders as the centrifugal and centripetal forces of globalization simultaneously draw us together and pull us apart. Under this view, neoliberalism and globalization go hand in hand, even as their effects may be highly variable in local contexts.

The figure of the neoliberal subject imagined by Nikolas Rose is powerful, particularly in the context of the emergence of the "psy" sciences, which he argues represent a problematic/flawed attempt to understand human actions scientifically, frequently in order to control them. This argument supports Foucault's notion that psychiatric patients and other subaltern people hold "subjugated knowledges," discounted and disbelieved in an enlightened society. At first glance,

Las Lomas appears to be merely another cog in Mexico's neoliberal wheel: neo-liberal economic reforms, begun in the presidency of Carlos Salinas de Gortari with the privatization of Telmex (the national telephone company) and other state-owned enterprises, has gradually become complete through various reforms, including the creation of Seguro Popular, which, despite the fact that it is a state-funded program, is premised on the ideals of personal responsibility and account-ability (Hayden 2007).

Dr. Mariana Garza and I sit in one of Las Lomas's many *consultorios*, its outpa-tient care offices. Mariana is not a psychiatrist; she is currently completing a spe-cialization in integrative medicine, a relatively new field currently being embraced by the Mexican government as part of its new health care approach. Integrative specialists are generalists; the training they receive is broad but centered around mental health, general medicine, and preventative care. Part of their training takes place at psychiatric facilities like Las Lomas, where they learn to assess, diagnose, and monitor psychiatric conditions.

On this particular day, Mariana is reviewing the case file of a patient, Simon. She has seen him regularly for the past few months and has come to the conclu-sion that his initial diagnosis, schizophrenia, made when he was hospitalized, is incorrect. Mariana has concluded that Simon is actually suffering from schizoaf-fective disorder, a different ailment. She adjusts his medication scheme, carefully jotting down medication names, dosages, and instructions.

"Okay, Don Simon," she says, "This one, you're going to take half of a tablet three times a day, okay? And this one is only at night. . . ." She continues down the list, explaining his new regimen, and then asks him to repeat it back. When she is satisfied that he understands which medications he needs to take when, she wishes him well and asks him to come back in a month.

Dr. Mariana bases her practice on ensuring her patient is self-sufficient enough to understand how to take his medication. During the visit, she also inquires about other social factors affecting the patient's life—his living situation, employment, and interpersonal relationships. The model of integrative medicine she is train-ing to provide assumes that the patient is a mostly rational being who will act in his own self-interest. By the same token, another interaction reveals how this phi-losophy is reconciled with the fact that patients are not, in fact, always or even mostly rational in their day-to-day lives.

For example, Imelda was a fifty-one-year-old woman whom Mariana had been treating for nearly six months. Imelda was having a difficult time. She lived with her son and his wife, who were angry with her because she was having a relationship with a married man. To Mariana's concern, though, she was also out of medication.

"I don't care if I have to live in a cardboard box," Imelda explained, "I want to live alone. My daughter-in-law locks herself up in her room and my son doesn't speak to me. I can't stand being there anymore."

"Okay," Mariana replied, "so what are you going to do? Do you have a plan? If you want to move out of your son's house, you have to have a plan, right?"

"Right . . ." Imelda replies, uneasily.

"What are you doing to recover? Part of recovering is to follow your medication regimen." This was clearly the "in" that Mariana was looking for.

"I've been taking my medication," Imelda protested.

"Read me your prescription, then."

Imelda looked at the piece of paper on the desk. "Well, it says. . . ." and faltered.

Mariana leaned forward, points to the prescription, and gently said, "You were going to reduce the dosage, right? By one drop, at night. And you haven't done so."

"I forget to read the paper. . . ." Imelda said in a wavering voice.

"You know what you want, Imelda," Mariana said with a sigh, "You can choose to recover, or you can choose to go back. You have to take your medication as prescribed. Imelda, this medication, you can't run out of it. You can't just stop taking it. If you run out, you have to come in and get more. But you have to follow a discipline. You have to make a commitment to yourself. And this is what you are going to do, starting tonight: you are only going to take five drops, okay? Just five. For two weeks. And in two weeks, you bring that down to four drops. And so on. Are you with me? It's all here in the prescription. It's your guide. Your *acordión*."[6]

Imelda was on liquid clonazepam, one of the most commonly prescribed anxiety medications in Mexico. It is a habit-forming medication; withdrawal can result in seizures and stopping can be dangerous. Mariana did not say this to Imelda; indeed, although clonazepam consumption is extremely common in Mexico, most people who take it are not aware of its potential for creating dependency or its dangerous withdrawal. Though Mariana emphasized to Imelda that she could not stop taking the medication, she did not explain to her that stopping the medication ran the risk of seizures or death.

By using admonishments such as *you can choose to recover, or you can choose to go back*, and *you have to make a commitment to yourself*, Mariana uses empowerment discourse to foster Imelda's sense of individual responsibility. Firmly within the boundaries of contemporary psychological and biomedical models, this approach places responsibility for recovery on Imelda herself. By the same token, Mariana's approach, though sympathetic to Imelda, also reveals vestiges of paternalism when she asks Imelda to read her script to her, or when she refers to Imelda's prescription as an *acordión*. Although Mariana's discourse attempts to foster individual responsibility and agency, noticeably absent in her instructions to Imelda is any information about the potentially serious side effects of benzodiazepine withdrawal. This practice is similar to the practice of *psicoeducación* described by Whitney Duncan (2017) in Oaxaca, though I never heard it referred to using that term. The purpose of psicoeducación is to encourage self-sufficiency and independence in the patients, an "emotion pedagogy" that plays an important role in psychological modernization in Mexico (3). However, even though Mariana voiced the self-actualizing logics of psicoeducación, the decision to wean Imelda from her medication is one-sided: Imelda has no input on her medication regimen. Despite the empowerment rhetoric, her only choices are whether or not to comply.

Two assumed subjectivities conflict in the Mexican health care system: one that looks to the state to guarantee the well-being of its population, and one that increasingly places this onus on individual actors, with a little help from the state. The drive to create self-acting neoliberal subjects at once reinforces the Mexican state's paternalistic logic toward its own citizenry. *Oportunidades*, the government direct remittances program for pregnant women and children, conditions these remittances on pregnant women receiving regular, state-sponsored prenatal care and attending regular parenting/nutrition/health classes; children's remittances are conditioned on regular school attendance regardless of performance (Smith-Oka 2013). This has resulted in a lower-income population that is more connected to state programming and ideologies than ever before, yet it holds a conflicted view of the state's effectiveness.

Cori Hayden (2007) notes that Seguro Popular betrays a neoliberal ideology in its premise that all Mexicans must take responsibility for becoming healthy citizen-subjects. By the same token, neoliberalism is not the only ideology circulating in Mexican public health. At the same time that the Mexican state fully embraced neoliberal economic policy, when Carlos Salinas de Gortari signed the North American Free Trade Agreement (NAFTA), the Zapatista rebellion of 1994 rose in direct opposition to it. The Zapatista rebellion called attention to the plight of indigenous people. This call resonated throughout the country. The Zapatista rebellion generated the national and international good will to eventually foster the passage of the *ley general de derechos lingüísticos de los pueblos indígenas* (general law of linguistic rights of indigenous peoples) in 2002, and the adoption of the tenets of *interculturalidad* (interculturality) into federal policies.

Interculturalidad is a popular framework adopted by several Latin American countries in the areas of services used by indigenous people. It refers to the interaction among various cultures from a strictly horizontal framework, a decolonizing strategy seeking to right previous wrongs done to indigenous and other subaltern peoples. The intercultural framework seeks to legitimize previously subjugated knowledges by integrating subaltern cultural elements into mainstream culture. Examples of these initiatives in Latin America include the incorporation of traditional medical practitioners such as midwives into allopathic care and accommodating certain cultural practices such as vertical birth (Llamas and Mayhew 2016) in public hospitals. In Mexico, intercultural education initiatives resulted in the creation of two indigenous intercultural universities in the Yucatan peninsula. The Indigenous Education System, a parallel public education system of elementary schools operating in communities the federal government has identified as indigenous, purportedly adopted intercultural principles in its pedagogy.

Intercultural principles center on the celebration and respect for traditional forms of life, specifically, in Mexico, for indigenous languages and cultures. In line with the 2002 Law of Linguistic Rights, all Mexican hospitals and court systems are required to hire interpreters and to provide services to people in their own languages. In the area of psychiatry, this model was successfully implemented in Guadalajara by Sergio Villaseñor Fajardo, a pioneer in the integration of indigenous worldviews into the practice of psychiatry (Villaseñor et al. 2003). In Mexico, an intercultural framework was included as a strategy in the health care portion of the 2007–2012 and 2013–2018 National Development Plans (Gobierno de la República 2013; Secretaría de Salud 2007–2012).

Like other institutions, Las Lomas is supposed to follow the tenets of interculturalidad. What this means in policy appears in a sign, *Lineamientos Interculturales* (Intercultural Guidelines), posted at the hospital entrance, and visible to anyone who comes in. Among the guidelines is point number three:

> Permita al paciente o a sus familiares comentar o realizar diferentes actividades relacionadas con sus creencias en un marco de respeto y escucha. *Evite burlarse, regañar, o prohibir* (utilizar amuletos, colocar imagines religiosas). En caso de contravenir una norma oficial, explicar claramente y con respeto la situación. Si usted *esta seguro* de que se trata de una practica nociva, explíquelo claramente y convenza al paciente.
>
> Allow the patient or their family to comment or carry out different activities related to their beliefs within a framework of respect and open-mindedness. *Avoid ridiculing, lecturing, or prohibiting* (using amulets, placing religious images). In case an official regulation precludes [a particular practice], explain it clearly and respectfully. If you *are sure* that the practice is harmful, explain this clearly and convince the patient. ("Lineamientos Interculturales," emphasis in original)

This point is the only one of the eight guidelines that is emphasized with bold lettering. This is quite telling. Doctors and other hospital staff are admonished to not ridicule, lecture, or prohibit patients and their families from engaging in certain practices. The fact that it is necessary to highlight this (and only this) admonishment with bold lettering suggests that these actions have been identified as an obstacle to the implementation of intercultural medicine. The admonishment that the hospital staff member *be sure* that a practice is harmful before somehow "convincing" the patient of this may point to an impulse to assume an inherent harmfulness in these unnamed practices.

There is something disingenuous and ambiguous about this admonishment. How is a doctor supposed to simply "convince" a patient that a particular practice is harmful? If regulation precludes a practice, is the staff member authorized

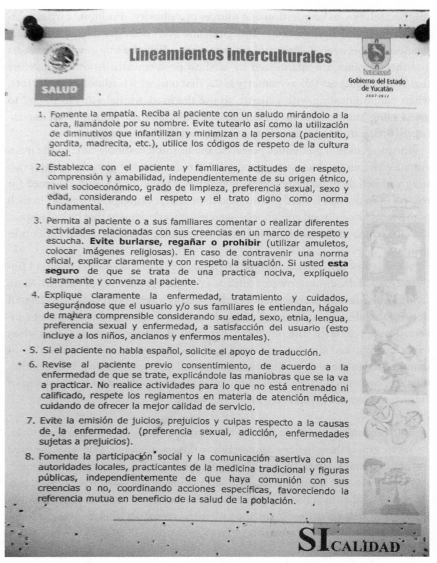

Lineamientos interculturales

Gobierno del Estado
de Yucatán
2007-2012

SALUD

1. Fomente la empatía. Reciba al paciente con un saludo mirándolo a la cara, llamándole por su nombre. Evite tutearlo así como la utilización de diminutivos que infantilizan y minimizan a la persona (pacientito, gordita, madrecita, etc.), utilice los códigos de respeto de la cultura local.

2. Establezca con el paciente y familiares, actitudes de respeto, comprensión y amabilidad, independientemente de su origen étnico, nivel socioeconómico, grado de limpieza, preferencia sexual, sexo y edad, considerando el respeto y el trato digno como norma fundamental.

3. Permita al paciente o a sus familiares comentar o realizar diferentes actividades relacionadas con sus creencias en un marco de respeto y escucha. **Evite burlarse, regañar o prohibir** (utilizar amuletos, colocar imágenes religiosas). En caso de contravenir una norma oficial, explicar claramente y con respeto la situación. Si usted **esta seguro** de que se trata de una practica nociva, explíquelo claramente y convenza al paciente.

4. Explique claramente la enfermedad, tratamiento y cuidados, asegurándose que el usuario y/o sus familiares le entiendan, hágalo de manera comprensible considerando su edad, sexo, etnia, lengua, preferencia sexual y enfermedad, a satisfacción del usuario (esto incluye a los niños, ancianos y enfermos mentales).

5. Si el paciente no habla español, solicite el apoyo de traducción.

6. Revise al paciente previo consentimiento, de acuerdo a la enfermedad de que se trate, explicándole las maniobras que se la va a practicar. No realice actividades para lo que no está entrenado ni calificado, respete los reglamentos en materia de atención médica, cuidando de ofrecer la mejor calidad de servicio.

7. Evite la emisión de juicios, prejuicios y culpas respecto a las causas de la enfermedad. (preferencia sexual, adicción, enfermedades sujetas a prejuicios).

8. Fomente la participación social y la comunicación asertiva con las autoridades locales, practicantes de la medicina tradicional y figuras públicas, independientemente de que haya comunión con sus creencias o no, coordinando acciones específicas, favoreciendo la referencia mutua en beneficio de la salud de la población.

SI CALIDAD

FIGURE 5. Yucatan Health Department Intercultural Guidelines poster on display at Las Lomas reception area. July 2012.

to prohibit, or merely expected to explain it? The very use of the word *evite* (avoid) weakens the admonishment that hospital staff not ridicule or lecture their patients about their practices. The use of the word *regañar* (scold) is also significant. "Regañar" reflects the paternalistic nature of medical practice in Mexico and other Latin American countries, where physicians have often been seen—and see themselves—as unquestionable sources of authority. "Prohibit" carries similar asymmetrical connotations. This guideline acknowledges the asymmetrical relationship between doctors and patients, particularly the way in which patients and their families are infantilized by medical professionals. Another guideline that seeks to address this asymmetry is the first one, which admonishes doctors, when communicating with patients, to use the more formal *usted* form and to avoid using "diminutives that infantilize and minimize the person," such as *pacientito* (little patient), *gordita* (fatty), and *madrecita* (little mother).

The intercultural guidelines posted in the hospital vestibule next to the main entrance encourage doctors and medical staff to *be respectful* of the language, practices and beliefs of patients and their families.[7] The concern with the need for respect from doctors toward patients and their families emerges repeatedly in each of the eight intercultural guidelines—a tacit acknowledgment that lack of respect has characterized the relationship between medical professionals and patients in the past.

Yet whether this admonishment carries into practice is another matter. I frequently heard the diminutive pacientito used by nurses referring to patients. More significantly, despite the posted notice, in my daily interactions with hospital staff none of the ideas or concerns of interculturality ever emerged as a topic of conversation or reference. The only time that cultural difference came up was when I specifically asked about it, and even then, doctors seemed either unfamiliar or uninterested in the premise of inclusion inherent in interculturality. While enthusiastic about rejecting the asylum model, Juan also pointed to the problem of culture and patient compliance inside the wards.

> Think about it, many of our patients do not sleep in beds, they sleep in hammocks. Yet we expect them to sleep comfortably in this environment. They might be used to eating beans and tortillas, and using their hands when they eat. Yet we expect them to eat a set menu and to use utensils. Some of the women may never wear anything other than their huipil and we force them—sometimes physically—to wear the hospital uniform. And then when they resist we label them as "uncooperative." (Field note excerpt, 2012)

This lack of intercultural awareness, however, is not because the psychiatrists are unaware of the lifeways of indigenous people in Yucatan—all the attending psychiatrists know that Maya people sleep in hammocks and wear huipil, as does any person born and raised in Yucatan. Additionally, Dr. Castro, the attending physician for male patients in the intensive care ward, lived in a remote Maya village as a young man; Dr. Pacheco, the IMSS psychiatrist, learned Yucatec Maya from his grandparents; and Dr. Tun is ethnically Maya, though she does not speak Mayan. Most nursing staff know or at the very least understand Yucatec Mayan. The only people unfamiliar with local culture and lifeways are the psychiatry residents, who come from all over the country to complete their specialization and stay for four years, and the integrative medicine residents, who also come from all over the country and rotate between various hospitals for a few months at a time.

So while the Mexican public health sector appears to embrace the principles of interculturalism—the "respectful, horizontal, and synergistic interaction of cultures" (Almaguer González, Vargas Vite, and García Ramírez 2014, 17) in its rhetoric—this embrace has not taken place in day-to-day practice. In the face of the decidedly *un*-intercultural practices occurring each day at Las Lomas, the sign is more a disingenuous attempt to acknowledge public policy than encouragement to engage in a practice that is decolonial at its core. The discordance of the sign and its ideals, and local practice, highlight the difficulties of transformation in a nation that remains overwhelmingly racist and mired in its own coloniality.

LAS LOMAS AS METAPHOR OF COLONIALITY

While interculturalidad is given plenty of lip service in public discourse, in practice—at least at Las Lomas—it amounts to little more than bilingual signage on the campus.[8] Some doctors and nurses are fluent in Yucatec Mayan, but the professional interpreters the hospital is supposed to have are nowhere to be found. As Juan points out, there is minimal acknowledgment of the fact that a large number of the patients who use psychiatric services at Las Lomas are indigenous. All patients are forced to wear a hospital uniform. For mestizas who wear huipil, this represents a violation, particularly in cases when their clothing is forcibly removed. For patients who are used to sleeping in hammocks, the old rubber mattresses of the hospital beds make it difficult to sleep comfortably. In the presence of mental illness, patients who cannot navigate these institutional demands are considered "uncooperative" and frequently subjected to worsening care. The existence of interculturalidad indicates a recognition of the problematic relationship between Mexican society and its indigenous people. It is an attempt to address this relationship in a way that does not result in the further oppression and marginalization of subaltern people and an implicit acknowledgement of past misdeed.

Moreover, this sign is a perfect symbol of the way in which coloniality is an enduring and defining characteristic of Mexican society, down to the microcosm of its institutions. As I noted in previous chapters, Mignolo (2011) refers to colonialism as the "darker side of Western modernity." When he says this, he means colonialism is constitutive of Western modernity (i.e., constructs of modernity reflecting the values of the Global North), that modernity *cannot* exist without colonialism because it is only through its colonial establishments—trade, slavery and its cognates, conquest, exploitation of natural resources—that it became possible. The coloniality of power is constitutive of modernity itself (Grosfoguel 2011a, 2011b). Some scholars argue for the possibility of alternative modernities (García Canclini 1989), of a way for postcolonial societies to construct their own modernities, a move Mignolo (2011) applauds and critiques at the same time: if colonialism is intricately intertwined with modernity, part of modernity, and constitutive of modernity, then all modernities are inherently colonial. And neo-liberalism, a defining economic and social ideology of our times, is colonialist modernity taken to an almost inconceivable extreme.

CAROLINA: Can you tell me why you are here?

INÉS: Well, because I was hearing voices.

CAROLINA: And when did you start hearing voices?

INÉS: When I was diagnosed with schizophrenia. But I'm not going to stuff myself with medication. I take it natural, if I feel good, I don't take it. The doctor gave me a prescription but my husband, he—the roles switched. I am my Viejo. But he isn't my husband, he's my son. I call my husband hijo.[9] Mi hijo [my son] is such a ladies' man. He's like a butterfly, going from flower to flower....

CAROLINA: Do you know where you are?

INÉS: A house, I think. A school.

CAROLINA: Do you see school desks? A blackboard?

INÉS: [Rubs her chest.] I have a lot of pain here. They say I have cancer, but I'm not the one with cancer, it's my sister. I'm not the one that has something wrong with me, it's my husband.

This exchange takes place between Carolina, a psychiatry resident, and Doña Inés, an older woman suffering from schizophrenia who is committed to the intensive care ward. The exchange is a simple assessment meant to elucidate whether the patient is properly oriented in space and time. Doña Inés is able to identify why she is at Las Lomas, but when she is asked if she knows where she is, she is unable to explain where she is. Her language is circular and confused—her husband, her son, her sister, and herself blend into one another as she speaks; her individual persona is elusive. These symptoms are not unusual for someone with Doña Inés's condition.

Luhrmann points out that schizophrenia, our "most troubling madness" (2016), is "a real and terrible disorder . . . that at its most severe has clearly recognizable features and is found in nearly every corner of the world" (1), and that previous anthropological treatises of the illness may have romanticized it. Luhrmann (Luhrmann and Marrow 2016) notes that the outcomes of patients with schizo-phrenia are highly contingent on their level of integration into society; in other words, patients with schizophrenia do better under social conditions where they are not turned into social pariahs but rather continue to be part of the family unit and participate in daily activities to the best of their abilities. These social condi-tions tend to occur in "developing nations," all of which are postcolonial societies.

This makes for an interesting paradox, as Yucatan, like Mexico, occupies the middle ground of being a contemporary postcolonial state struggling to "become modern." Inés's blended persona may have no place inside the wards of Las Lomas, but what her life is like when she is home, surrounded by her family, is something I was unable to ascertain. Inside the wards, Inés's insistence that she takes a "natural" approach, opting to not take her medication if "she feels fine," is unacceptable; the first line of psychiatric assessment is to ascertain the orientation of a patient in space, time, and person. Does the patient know where she is? Does she know what day of the week it is? What year? What time of day? Does she know *who she is*? What is interesting in this line of questioning is the underlying concern that the patient be connected with "reality," that the patient be rational enough to know what these constructs (orientation in space, time, and person) are. It may be of particular relevance that time, a social construct with deep roots in industrialization and the management of workers (Engels 1993), is the first one listed. The second, place, is a nod at the importance of the institution, and agreement that the location in which the patient finds herself is a place of healing. Equally important is that the patient's own individual personhood—a bounded, stable, unquestionably modern self—is reaffirmed. Agreement on these three things—time, place, and self—is a prerequisite to any other progress made. In the exchange, Inés has failed the first line of psychiatric assessment: Carolina will now note on her record that she is oriented in neither space, nor time, nor person. She will remain in the intensive care ward until she can answer those questions to the physicians' satisfaction.

Las Lomas as the materialization of psychiatric care may thus be read as overt coloniality—the only acceptable reality is the one in which the day of the week is Monday, the time is morning, the place is the acute ward of a psychiatric ward, and the self is Inés Vallado, sixty-seven years old, from the town of Ticul. There is, however, nuance in this picture. Las Lomas is not simply a place where beautiful minds arrive to be disciplined and repressed into a modern semblance of normal. To return to Dr. Vasquez's interaction with Dora, patients themselves have different beliefs and attitudes toward Las Lomas, some of which can be problematic.

On the morning I first met Lina in 2012, Dr. Tun groaned as she picked up the clipboard listing the overnight admissions. "Not her again!" she said, when she read her name. Lina was in her mid-twenties at the time, and she was a college graduate with a degree in a mental health field. Lina seemed to be a thorn in Dr. Tun's side. Her thick patient file revealed she had been committed at least once a year for the last four years. Dr. Tun had been her attending psychiatrist for three of those years. Lina was brought in that morning, and I observed Dr. Tun interview her. The interview itself was uneventful. Lina came in, sat down, yawned through Dr. Tun's basic questions—did she know who she was? Where she was? What day of the week it was? She responded correctly, if sleepily. As occurred with her prior stays, Lina was committed following a suicide attempt, this time with clonazepam. Having answered her questions, Dr. Tun asked Lina if she was tired and would rather speak with her later, to which Lina readily agreed. "We will talk tomorrow, then," Dr. Tun decided.

When the interview was over, and Lina returned to the ward, Dr. Tun let out a sigh. She turned to me. "I have to treat her," she explained, "I *have* to. Legally. Otherwise, I wouldn't. Lina and I . . . there is so much transference and counter-transference. I feel my own tension rising just knowing she's here. She manipulates everyone around her." Caught between a rock and a hard place, knowing she should not be responsible for Lina's care, but having no option to transfer her to another psychiatrist, Dr. Tun finally decided to turn over Lina's day-to-day care to her psychiatry residents, allowing them to assess and make recommendations based on her progress. They recommended she be moved to the long-term ward as soon as possible. When she heard that she was being transferred, Lina broke down in tears and cut herself. "The doctor only sees you once a day there," she wept. "Here they see you three times a day." She wanted to be seen three times a day, she objected, not once.

As she went through her file, Dr. Tun explained that Lina liked to use her knowledge of psychology to describe and emulate symptoms that she knew would result in her commitment. The suicide attempt that had brought her in to Las Lomas this time was not the first. The psychiatry interns who closely monitored Lina claimed they would often watch her shift behaviors when she thought she was not being watched—chatting with the other patients in the ward, making jokes, laughing—and instantly shift her demeanor in the presence of the doctors. In Dr. Tun's words, "Lina is a sane woman who wants to be treated as if she were psychotic. She *wants* to be tied up, she *wants* to be put in isolation, she *wants* to be sedated. She's not psychotic. Her actions are logical. They just don't follow *our* logic."

According to Dr. Tun, Lina attempted to manipulate the institution into fulfilling her desire to be treated as though she were insane. As Dr. Tun used the institution to further pressure Lina into complying—by putting her in isolation, by minimizing her contact with doctors, by unsuccessfully attempting to transfer her into another ward—Lina appeared to get exactly what she wanted. Evident in the interactions between Dr. Tun and Lina is an underlying moral register: for Dr. Tun, Lina presents a challenge and a problem because she "wants to be" treated as though she were insane. Lina's desire to be ill counters Dr. Tun's view that patients need to recover from their illness, and recovery looks like a return to a productive, socially responsible life.

Lina confounds the institution because she wants to be inside it, albeit somewhat differently from Dora, Dr. Vasquez's patient, for whom Las Lomas represents an escape from her difficult life. Claudina, who I introduced in chapter 2, had been hospitalized at Las Lomas in 2008 following a psychotic break accompanied by a suicide attempt. Claudina and I got to know each other over several weeks as she participated in small-group therapy sessions as part of Las Lomas's suicide prevention program, *La Esperanza*. Claudina was remarkable in several ways, most notably that even though she came from a working-class family and had not completed high school, she was among the very few patients who seemed to perfectly understand what I was doing in Las Lomas. She frequently referred to the "the book I was writing" and my role as an observer in the hospital. Claudina was a philosopher—she thought deeply about things, her own life conditions, the state of society. During her time at the hospital, she would come in, wearing the hospital uniform, an ugly blue or green smock, her long black hair in a French braid. She would smile, participate enthusiastically in the session, share some of her newest insights. Eventually, her symptoms under control and newly diagnosed with bipolar depression, Claudina went home.

A few weeks after she left Las Lomas, she attended La Esperanza's outpatient group therapy session. A stylist by trade, Claudina looked stunning: wearing jeans and a tucked-in green button-up blouse hanging loosely on her petite frame, her hair now loose and perfectly blow-dried, and wearing makeup, she was almost unrecognizable from the plain woman I had met on the ward. During the session, several participants who, like Claudina, had found themselves committed to Las Lomas following a suicide attempt, shared their experiences dealing with the aftermaths of their suicide attempts. Finally, she raised her hand to speak.

> I remember. . . . I shut myself in, I felt trapped, I worked twice or three times as hard helping my mother. This produced so much anxiety, and my parents did not allow me to continue my studies and this was my second depression. Then my parents realized how sad I was, and this was my third depression. And then I wore my knees out (working out) . . . so in July I tried to kill myself. I wanted to die. I thought, all that ever happens to me is sadness. . . . Being here [inside Las Lomas] is like being in a monastery. We find silence, and nature. The sounds are clearer. I realized that I was causing great harm to my parents and my younger siblings. I will not open doors that I cannot close. (Field note excerpt, November 2008)

While there is much to unpack in Claudina's story—she became an influential figure in my early work in Merida—it is in her description of Las Lomas as a monastery that we can clearly see the powerful persistence of the figure of the mental institution-as-asylum, despite the state's best efforts to move away from it. Strikingly, the first hospitals in Yucatan were created and operated by Franciscan friars, making the monastery comparison especially apt. Claudina's evocation of *silence* and *nature* as bringing her clarity she did not have before further reifies the model. Having had the opportunity to interact with Claudina from the time she was committed in July to this meeting in November, I witnessed her journey. Claudina's worldview was heavily influenced by her spirituality; that the *sounds were clearer* inside the ward further reifies her view of the hospital as a sanctuary.

Ironically, Claudina's evocation of the monastery, which is so closely connected to Yucatan's colonial history, represents a different subjectivity than the neoliberal autonomous citizen Las Lomas attempts to rehabilitate. Yet one can see how the space of the ward, even though it is a strictly secular space lacking any religious symbols or paraphernalia, could be construed in this light: the long-term area of the hospital, also known as "the garden," is an open space. One-story buildings hold dormitories and medical examination rooms, but the common areas are all outdoors, in a garden full of tall shade trees and fragrant flowers connected by walkways with benches. The garden is worlds away from the horrors of the acute ward, where patients are locked indoors in stifling conditions. The garden can easily become a sanctuary to a person who is looking for one.

Thus, the coloniality of power at Las Lomas can be identified on multiple levels, and it must be understood in the context of Mexico's own status as a modern state struggling under the weight of its own inescapable coloniality. On a broad level, the explicit mission of Las Lomas is the rehabilitation of its patients into neoliberal subjects capable of engaging in enough self-care that they can function in society outside of the institution. However, on a second level, the institution is, at least rhetorically, obligated to respect the tenets of interculturalidad and respect and honor the cultural diversity of its client population. Thus, the mandate to rehabilitate neoliberal subjects is tempered by the mandate to honor and respect—*in a horizontal manner*—the language and traditions of the local population. On a third level, the institution must also deal with the fact that regardless of language or traditions, patients come to Las Lomas with individual motives, beliefs, and agendas. Many of these patients are experiencing psychosis and suffering from a variety of debilitating ailments frequently compounded by obstacles in their immediate social environments, aggravating their symptoms. At the same time, the institution is plagued by shortages, corruption, and its own precarious place within Mexico's government health care schema, subject to the whims of local politics, as I will explore in chapter 5.

When Mignolo says that coloniality is the darker side of Western modernity, he points out the inescapability of coloniality from modernity: it is impossible to be modern without being colonial. In the contemporary neoliberal regime, the descendants of the European colonizers of Mexico continue to profit from their allegiances with the developed economies of Europe and the United States, as income inequality reentrenches itself. The modern individual conceptualized at the heart of neoliberal subjectivity—rational, self-serving, self-governing—comes up against other kinds of personhoods found in societies full of Others. As I show in the following chapters, at Las Lomas, multiple personhoods frustrate neoliberal models of health care and governance in general at every turn. Seeing the contemporary Mexican state and its institutions as the messy result of a very imperfect and flawed attempt by colonized minds to create colonizing institutions based on the unquestioned premise that modern values of the Global

North are superior or desirable has resulted in institutions that crumble under the weight of an "every-man-for-himself" Mexican culture of corruption.

This is what makes writing about subjectivity, neoliberalism, and the state so difficult. It may well be the case that there is no quintessential Euro-American, neoliberal society full of self-actualizing, neoliberal subjects. Where Foucault gives us a traditionally European narrative of the progression from the asylum model to the biomedicalization of psychiatric care, the disaster of Las Lomas is clear evidence that the project of modernity in Mexico is destined for failure because so long as Mexico pursues modernity, it will continue to reproduce the colonial matrix of power. It cannot do otherwise. Contrary to what many Mexican intellectuals bemoan, Mexico is not trying to be modern. It *is* modern. It cannot be anything other than its own fractured, colonial modernity.

5 · NEGOTIATING TRUTH IN THE PSYCHIATRIC ENCOUNTER

Truth is not only the outcome of construction, but of contestation...
truth... is always enthroned by acts of violence.
—Nikolas Rose (1996, 55)

The diagnosis is the icing. It's what's underneath that's the cake.
—Enrique, advanced psychiatry resident, Las Lomas

SESIÓN CLÍNICA

Eva, the young chemist introduced in chapter 1 who had found herself committed to Las Lomas, fascinated Dr. Tun and her residents.[1] Her story was remarkable perhaps because Eva herself was a remarkable woman: very few girls from faraway coastal villages with scarce resources finished degrees in the hard sciences and became laboratory employees at the Merida research center. Her psychotic break, the circumstances surrounding it, and her internal struggle with her perceived mission to lift her family above their financial hardships drew the attention of many psychiatry residents in the hospital. Thus, Eva's case was selected for *sesión clínica*, a clinical case-study session held once a week where a particular case was presented to the entire hospital staff. While these sessions are really mandatory only for the Las Lomas residents, they are attended by other hospital staff, particularly those in psychology and social work.

Sesión clínica sessions consist of a written report produced by a psychiatric resident and a series of oral presentations made by the same resident, a psychologist, and a social worker. These sessions are generally very interesting because they feature a truly interdisciplinary way of processing and understanding particular clinical cases. The exercise is meant to help residents understand the team-based, multifaceted nature of psychiatric treatment. Psychiatrists present the patient's clinical history—including circumstances surrounding their mother's pregnancy and birth, considered standard part of any clinical history (and potentially indicative of complications such as fetal brain injury), psychiatric diagnosis, and ensuing treatment. The psychologist presents the results of particular psychometric tests administered and discusses her experiences in treating the patient; usually she takes a psychodynamic approach that considers the patient's inner life and struggles. Finally, a social worker discusses the patient's immediate social environment, including results from home visits, interpersonal relationships, and socioeconomic context.

Enrique, an advanced resident in the same cohort as Ana, whose interaction with Dr. Patrón is described in chapter 4, had volunteered to lead Eva's case study. He stood before the sparsely attended room, with about eleven people in the audience, and began reciting Eva's clinical history. He read from a slide show he had prepared, attempting to present a full portrait of Eva by recounting the circumstances of her birth, her early childhood, age at sexual initiation, and life experiences including her father's death and career trajectory, before beginning to describe the circumstances surrounding her admission, treatment, and release from Las Lomas. During this time, I knew that the case presented was Eva's, because Dr. Tun had told me her case had been selected for session and because I was familiar with her case, but her name was left out of the presentation and she was simply referred to as "the patient."

In his description of Eva's stay, Enrique included information on her daily treatments, laboratory test results, and medication regimen. When it came to describing Eva's symptoms, he noted that Eva had experienced "poorly structured magical-religious delusions," without going into further detail.

Once Enrique had concluded his presentation, Eva's psychologist, Diana, stood up. Diana's presentation also included a slide show, where she projected images of Eva and her mother's psychological screenings. "The patient is a woman with above average intelligence," Diana explained to the audience, projecting side-by-side self-representations that Eva and her mother had drawn. Both women had drawn themselves holding umbrellas, getting rained on, except in Eva's picture, the umbrella did not help, and she portrayed herself as drenched under the rain. The audience murmured, fascinated by the childlike drawings, as Diana explained how the presence of trees in the images indicated Eva's desire to reach high for success.

When Diana completed her presentation, Adriana, a social worker, took her turn. Adriana explained that she had gotten to know the family only superficially, but she had been able to conduct a home visit and speak with a few family members. Projecting Eva's family tree, including her mother and siblings, Adriana described the dysfunctional family dynamics, the legal squabbles, and fighting that had proven so stressful to Eva.

"The patient has returned home," Adriana concluded, "but we have another home visit planned to ensure her well-being and make sure she continues to be supported."

By now, nearly half an hour had transpired since the beginning of the session. The session opened to questions from the audience. The residents asked questions about symptoms, and finally Dr. Tun, in her role as a teacher, stood before the room. "Very well, doctors," she said, "what is your diagnosis?"

Carolina, who had assisted Dr. Tun in treating Eva, spoke first. "Well, I think she suffered from an acute psychotic episode, but I can't find another diagnosis. When it comes to Axis II[2] she has no personality disorder, though she has certain traits—we know she's a perfectionist. In Axis III, all she has is that allergy she had, but she's not sick. In Axis IV she has her family problems and money troubles. In Axis V, I'd give her a 51–60, because she did have problems at work."

Ana, the advanced resident I met while working in the emergency room, spoke next. "I agree with the doctor, that we are dealing with a transitory acute, polymorphous psychotic disorder. There doesn't seem to be any other symptomatology, though a Skinner test might be a good idea. I don't think she has any Axis II personality disorders, but she does have some traits, and we said, she's not sick, ruling out an Axis III diagnosis. Her problems with her family and her boyfriends are part of Axis IV. Personally, in Axis V I would give her a 41–50 at admission and a 71–80 at release."

Dr. Tun nodded. "Okay, very good. Would you modify her treatment?"

Carolina spoke first. "Well, the symptoms remitted, so I think she can continue her medication treatment and combine it with therapy."

Ana shrugged. "Personally, I think her admission could have been avoided, as this is something that is going to mark her [socially]. I think she could have come in, been treated with another antipsychotic—my personal preference—and [then she should have been] sent home, for follow up outside the institution. It would have been better for the patient if she had not been admitted to the hospital, and I don't think she needed to be admitted. Her case could have been handled differently."

Dr. Tun nodded again. "How would you have dealt with Eva's dysfunctional family situation? How would you focus your therapeutic interventions?"

Again, Ana shrugged. "I would try to talk to her about what she thinks about what happened, particularly how she conceives of failure, and whether she considers ending up here a failure."

Dr. Tun raised an eyebrow, vaguely annoyed. "And her treatment?"

"The treatment worked. She should stay on it. I would just add an antidepressant."

"Which one?"

"Whichever, it doesn't matter," replied Ana.

Dr. Tun finished the session by having Enrique share his own diagnostic rationale. Enrique, projecting his rationale on the screen, came to a similar conclusion: brief psychotic disorder in Axis I, some compulsive personality traits, but insufficient to warrant a personality disorder in Axis II, a sulfonamide allergy in Axis III, problems within her primary support network, living alone and having insufficient income in Axis IV, and finally, in Axis V, a score of 11–20 at admission (meaning a high probability of harm to self or others) and 71–80 at release (meaning high functionality with mild, passing symptoms).

At the end of the session, Dr. Tun and I walked from the air-conditioned classroom space back toward the acute ward. "Did you notice," Dr. Tun asked me, "that neither of the residents suggested taking Eva off her antipsychotics, even though the diagnosis was that this was a transitory episode? Ana suggested putting her on *more* medication!" she scoffed.

"I did notice," I said, "does this upset you?"

"It's always about pharmaceuticals," she said irritably. "Their training is leading them to conclude that pharmaceutical treatment is the norm, that it is acceptable and desirable to put patients on long-term regimens of antipsychotics and antidepressants without first ascertaining whether or not this is actually necessary. For example, look at Eva. Eva had one psychotic episode that remitted almost immediately, after a lifetime without any kind of psychiatric symptoms. Why keep her indefinitely on an antipsychotic? Why add an antidepressant to the mix without even suggesting therapy or, better yet, addressing the family dysfunction that triggered the break in the first place? But this is considered standard practice now."

Later that day, I had the opportunity to congratulate Enrique on a job well done during his presentation. "It's just a really interesting case, you know?" he said. "The patient had so much going on inside. The diagnosis is the icing. It's what's underneath that's the cake."

Enrique had been genuinely interested by Eva's story. He was struck by her sudden psychosis and its equally sudden remission, her struggle to fulfill a mission to help her dysfunctional family out of poverty, her determination as a woman from a small village to live alone in a big city in a conservative society where few women—even the ones from Merida—leave their parents' homes before marriage. For Enrique, the pleasurable work of psychiatry went deeper than the diagnosis; rather, it was in focusing on the psyche and inner working of the brain. As Luhrmann (2000) observes in her analysis of the training of psychiatric residents in the United States, by the end of residency, diagnosis has long ceased being the primary goal of psychiatric work.

The opportunity to directly observe clinical sessions allowed me yet another moment to witness the ways that psychiatrists and other hospital staff frame and explain mental illness and individual patients. Although what I have just presented is an outline of what transpired, the discussion portion of the event provided the opportunity for residents, doctors, psychologists, and other staff to share their thoughts, first impressions, and make off-the-cuff remarks in a more informal environment. These were some of the comments made during the informal discussion portion of the session.

"Well she told me she was committed because she went to the beach and her mother thought she was going to kill herself." (Diana, psychologist)

"She showed up here, wearing an evening gown in the middle of the day, completely inappropriate to the time and place, complaining of nervios, three nights before her date of admission. We could have started antipsychotics then." (Ana, advanced resident)

"She seems to have obsessive-compulsive traits, doesn't she?" (Daniela, first-year resident)

"She keeps talking about this mission her father set out for her before he died. She talks about her father as if he were a saint, but he drank himself to death! The man was a hopeless alcoholic! The family's dysfunction probably starts there." (Carolina, first-year resident)

"Missions, missions. This young woman imposes so many missions on herself. Her ego is completely fractured, with only these missions holding it together. She broke under the stress because she is the healthiest member of her family." (Dr. Tun)

Each of these participants shares an impression of Eva's case that is not part of the formal diagnostic process or her medical file, yet conversations such as these form an important part of the psychiatric encounter and serve to frame how practitioners think of their patients and mental illness more broadly. Patients, too, are active agents in their own care, even when their agency is restricted and contingent on the limitations imposed by the institution. In the analysis of these psychiatric encounters—encounters between providers, or between patients and providers—the operationalization of the colonial matrix of power can come into view. Dr. Tun's criticism of the biomedicalization of psychiatric training and its shortcomings, of which observations have been made by anthropologists working in other settings (Luhrmann 2000; Kleinman 1980; Jenkins 2015), is one such segue, but there are others. The concerns expressed by psychiatrists channel the guiding ethos of Las Lomas as a neoliberal medical institution. A consideration of the ways in which psychiatrists and patients interact with each other is one way to see the functioning of psychiatric power in the colonial matrix of power. In this chapter, I explore multiple psychiatric encounters between patients and their doctors. I argue that the colonial matrix of power, as an intricate web of social interactions, is visible in these encounters, as doctors and patients negotiate the meaning of truth and orient themselves—toward each other, in physical space, and in reality.

PSYCHIATRIC POWER IN THE COLONIAL
MATRIX OF POWER

On a hot, muggy day in July 2012, Dr. Pacheco, the IMSS psychiatrist, and his patient, Manuela, sat across from each other in his office at Las Lomas. Manuela, who had been brought to Las Lomas in a psychotic state as an unknown person, had finally responded to medication and had become coherent enough to interview. Dr. Pacheco, who became her attending psychiatrist once her identity and insurance status had been confirmed, invited me to sit in on his daily evaluation with her.

DR. PACHECO: Manuela, are you bothered by the fact that sometimes I, that I might doubt some of the things you tell me? I feel that not everything you tell me is true. There are many things that are true, but there are others that are not. Do you mind that sometimes I don't believe everything you tell me?

MANUELA: Do you think I am a liar?

DR. PACHECO: No. Well, it's not that you are a liar—

MANUELA: I understand. When I tell you things about myself, you don't believe it all, just about half?

DR. PACHECO: More or less half. Exactly. I believe part of it. But when you tell me you studied five degrees, it seems difficult. I mean, not impossible, but—

MANUELA: Okay, let me keep just one. I studied—

DR. PACHECO: Haha, yes, I like that, that's right.

MANUELA: I studied to be a handcraft teacher.

DR. PACHECO: Okay, that's more like it. It's more believable. (Field recording)

Although I will analyze this exchange in greater depth, this passage raises important questions about psychiatric diagnosis, treatment, and doctor-patient relationships. However, the most important question emerging from this exchange pertains to truth. Dr. Pacheco asks Manuela if she is concerned that he does not believe she is telling the truth.

Elizabeth Davis refers to deception, especially deception in therapeutic settings, as a "pragmatic mode of sociality" (2010, 73). Davis (2010, 2012) observes that the history of psychiatry in Greece is more than a story of governmentality and neoliberalism, but also a story of the relationships and collaborations between practitioners and patients and the limits of those collaborations. This is not so different from the one in Mexico, where (as I discuss in chapter 4) deception, noncompliance, corruption, and transparency are all components of the Mexican national experience and Mexico's conversation with itself about its future in the twenty-first century. According to Davis, deception is a "refraction of responsibility through a constitutive opacity in intimate ethical relations" (2010, 136). In other words, suspicions of deception held by practitioners are necessary to the therapeutic relationship and help constitute it. "If self-presentation, on the part of the patient, and diagnosis, on the part of the therapist, are distancing maneuvers by which each take on a conventional role in the clinical encounter, then lying is the maneuver by which a more intimate, if antagonistic, relation can be recuperated from this distance in a mutual act of counter-transparency" (133).

In this chapter, I examine interactions at Las Lomas to engage three important regimes at play in daily operation: truth, negotiation, and orientation. In my time doing fieldwork at Las Lomas, between my work with Esperanza and my observations in the inpatient and outpatient services, I was privy to hundreds of interactions between patients and doctors in various settings. I was able to observe the socialization of medical residents into the work of diagnosing and treating patients. I participated in informal conversations between doctors and hospital staff. In this chapter, I consider what these interactions can tell us about the relationship between patient and provider, about the creation, reproduction, and hierarchical emplacement of relationships, and about the work of "making" doctors and patients in a highly problematic, deeply troubled therapeutic setting. These processes operationalize the colonial matrix of power created in the complex web of structure and relationships I describe in chapter 4. The interactions I describe are complex events characterized by negotiation and deception in ways that are ultimately connected, either through reinforcement or resistance, to neoliberal governance. Specifically, I introduce the notion of orientation as an interactive process of negotiation at Las Lomas and argue that this notion is central to the production and reproduction of hierarchies of care inside its wards.

Like other hospitals in Mexico and around the world, anyone who walks into Las Lomas can see a prominently displayed Patients' Bill of Rights. In addition to the right to "receive adequate medical care" and to "be treated with dignity and respect," users of Las Lomas services also have the right to "receive clear and true information," to make "free decisions about their care," and, most importantly, the right to "give or refuse validly informed consent." Patients' Bills of Rights like the one at Las Lomas are predicated on the idea that patients are and should be rational human beings capable of understanding their options and making informed decisions about their medical care—hallmarks of neoliberal subjectivity (Rose 1996). Although one could argue that a challenge faced by any neoliberal medical system is precisely the fact that it will always treat a population that will fall short of its ideal of rationality and self-actualization, the acute psychiatric patient presents a particular challenge.

Madness presents a paradox to liberal individualism. If *irrationality* is the fundamental symptom of the psychiatric patient, how can an institution treat its inherently irrational patients in a way that does not violate rights that were envisioned to be held by rational individuals? How does the institution treat a subject who violates its underlying ethos? In her ethnography of psychiatric reform

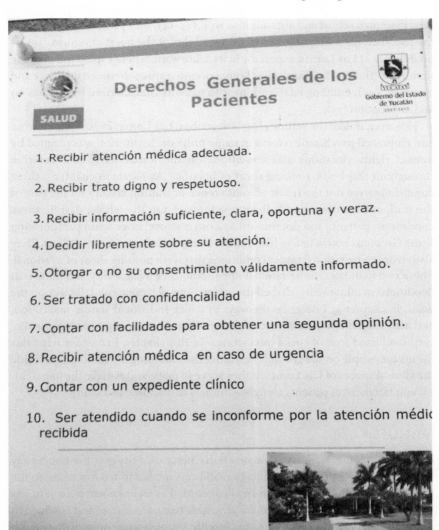

FIGURE 6. Yucatan Health Department Patients' Bill of Rights poster on display at Las Lomas reception area. July 2012.

in Thrace, Greece, Elizabeth Davis (2012) engages with this conundrum through the concept of responsibility. Psychiatric reform in Greece, like psychiatric reform in Mexico, is premised on political (neo)liberalism, humanitarian preoccupations with human rights and dignity, and psychodynamic and pharmaceutical treatment. When patients are enrolled in psychiatric treatment "by an agency other than their own robust and autonomous will" (13–14), they present a challenge to the foundational ethics of personal responsibility at the heart of reform. This is no different at Las Lomas, especially in its acute ward, where I spent much of my time. As in Thrace, clinicians at Las Lomas occupy a space "between guidance and coercion" (14), building relationships with patients characterized by persuasion and negotiation (15).

However, unlike the settings Davis describes, Las Lomas in 2008 and in 2012 had embraced psychiatric reform in name only: the institution was plagued by human rights violations and conditions on the wards were, as I describe throughout this book, nothing short of horrific.[3] As I state in chapter 1, these conditions were not the result of indifference or wanton cruelty on the part of the staff, at least none that I directly witnessed. On the whole, despite these conditions, patients and doctors at Las Lomas strove, once again paraphrasing Boris Grebenschikov, to live like human beings in inhumane conditions. They also strove to be rational under conditions that were nothing short of irrational. These two mandates, to be rational in conditions of irrationality and human in conditions of inhumanity, shaped the interactions of patients and doctors on the ward. In chapter 4, I describe the ways in which individual action, institution, and national policy interweave to form the colonial matrix of power, a contradictory, conflicted web of social interactions. In this chapter, I consider what this means for people on the ground. I consider the unfolding of relationships inside the clinical spaces of Las Lomas as they serve to make and remake the hierarchical emplacement of patients along the borders of madness and sanity.

MANUELA

Manuela was found wandering the streets in Chetumal, a city over five hours away from Merida. She had no identification and was unable to tell her name to the police officers who found her. She was committed as an unknown person to Las Lomas acute ward, where she remained, unable to communicate and confined to a solitary observation room, for nearly a month. Manuela spent most of that month screaming incoherently, spitting at doctors and nurses, or tied to her bed, sedated. Without any way of verifying her identity, there was no family to contact. Without drug testing strips, at first there was no way of knowing if her behavior was drug induced. One Monday, about a month after she first arrived, I came in to the hospital to discover that Manuela had become responsive over the weekend. She was able to tell the hospital staff her name, and her family was finally contacted.

After she finally revealed her name, and hospital workers contacted her family, Las Lomas staff learned that she had been living in Cancun and working at a supermarket. Her family claimed that her delusions had been triggered by the death of her only child eight years prior. She had been missing for several months before she was found in Chetumal. When I interviewed her, Manuela was adamant she had never lost her sense of reality:

MANUELA: I have never lost my sanity, even though they have drugged me.
BEATRIZ: You have always been completely aware of everything going on around you?
MANUELA: Yes, I was coherent. I remember when they brought me in. And I am still coherent, no matter what they do.

As far as Manuela was concerned, the police who had found her wandering the streets in Chetumal had targeted her unfairly and brought her to Las Lomas for no good reason. In her interview, which took place after her conversation with Dr. Pacheco, Manuela conceded nothing: she made it clear that she did not trust Dr. Pacheco or anyone else in the hospital. She understood, however, that she needed to satisfy him in order to leave Las Lomas.

The elicitation of a rational neoliberal subject is the ultimate goal for psychiatrists and other staff at Las Lomas. Modern Mexican psychiatry, which developed in parallel to the evolution of psychiatry in Europe and the United States, moved away from the asylum model, where psychiatric institutions were essentially homes for the insane (Foucault 1988a, 1988b), and moved toward biological psychiatry and the pharmaceutical management of mental illness (Lakoff 2005). This shift was predicated on the notion that psychiatric patients should be rehabilitated to return or become productive members of society rather than to be housed in asylums. The ideal that users of state medical services should be rational, empowered individuals remains strong in neoliberal Mexico. Although the creation of Seguro Popular guarantees universal access to medical care for the poorest uninsured Mexicans, Hayden (2007) notes that the Mexican federal government's rationale for the plan, which seeks to engage its target population through a combination of education, preventative medicine, and small financial contributions from participants, is premised on the idea of individual responsibility, the foundation of neoliberal personhood (Barry, Osborne, and Rose 1996).

In the interaction presented at the beginning of this chapter, Dr. Pacheco pushes a sensitive question. When Manuela first emerged from the deeply psychotic stage she was in at admission, she made the unlikely claim that she held five *licenciaturas*.[4] She also claimed to be a Canadian citizen, to work for Interpol, and to be fluent in Spanish, English, French, and Yucatec Mayan. By the time Dr. Pacheco posted this question to Manuela—*Are you bothered by the fact that I may not believe everything you say?*—Manuela and Dr. Pacheco had established a relationship over weeks of treatment. This was the first time he attempted to question the factuality of her claims. He did so, however, by reifying her position as an autonomous subject: *Are you bothered?* He asks her a subjective question about how his viewpoint might make her feel.

This initial approach results in the first negotiation: Manuela asks Dr. Pacheco if he thinks she is a liar (does he think she is deliberately or maliciously misleading him?), and he answers, decisively, no. Once that is settled, *she is not a liar*, she offers: *So you believe about half of what I say*? And Dr. Patrón gives some ground: yes, something like that. He concedes that she may in fact be telling the truth: *it seems difficult. Not impossible, but difficult.* Then she concedes as well: *let me keep one.* Dr. Pacheco does not hide pleasure at this concession, but laughs in delight— *yes, I like that . . . it's more believable.*

The "really" real truth of Manuela's story isn't at stake. Dr. Pacheco is not concerned with whether Manuela is telling him the truth. He may not even be concerned with whether Manuela believes she is telling him either truth (five degrees or one?). Dr. Pacheco's delight is with Manuela's ability to negotiate with him an acceptable narrative, a narrative that is *believable*. And at the heart of this negotiation is the fact that the basis of effective negotiation is diplomacy: the finding of a common ground that is possible only between two rational subjects. Manuela is not conceding the truth of her narrative. She is conceding that her narrative must change, and she is thus acting as a rational neoliberal subject.[5] Having made this concession, Dr. Pacheco notes that Manuela is making progress, the first step toward her eventual release.

MARIBEL

I suppressed a gasp when I first met Maribel. As she hobbled in, cradling her arm, we could see, clearly, that she had been badly hurt. Deep cuts on her head had been sewn back together with a multitude of stitches. Her knees and elbows showed raw, painful scrapes, as though she had been dragged. Her hospital gown was too large for her, and fell off her shoulder, revealing two large angel wings tattooed on her back. Now in her early thirties, Maribel had been diagnosed with schizophrenia ten years prior. This was the sixth time she had been committed to Las Lomas. Dr. Tun reviewed Maribel's file as she tried to make sense of her case. Maribel had a small house on a plot of land she shared with her mother, but the two families—Maribel and her two children, and her mother, who had a spouse and other children at home—were constantly bickering. In addition to schizophrenia, Maribel had a history of substance abuse. Recently, her relationship with her stepfather had been deteriorating, and things had finally come to a head.

MARIBEL: My mom has that man in my house, and he's constantly hitting me.
DR. TUN: Why does he hit you?
MARIBEL: He doesn't approve of me, he doesn't like me. If I want to bring something to my children and they're at my house, he makes fun of me. He raped me three months ago!
DR. TUN: Does your mother know about this?

MARIBEL: She's aware of everything. She knows I'm trying to get that man out of my house, but she doesn't react.

DR. TUN: So the wounds on your head, Maribel, how did they happen?

MARIBEL: He did this to me, with a rock. He hits me all the time.

DR. TUN: Are you married?

MARIBEL: I'm divorced. But my ex-husband doesn't help us in any way.

DR. TUN: So how do you survive?

MARIBEL: I panhandle on the street. I paid for my little house through prostitution.

Maribel lived a difficult life, resorting to panhandling (begging) and occasional sex work to provide for her children and herself. It was unclear whether she was able to access medication to treat her schizophrenia, but she did not appear to take it regularly. Her husband had abandoned her after her initial diagnosis, leaving her to depend on her mother for help. Her illness and substance abuse—primarily through the misuse of paint thinner and similar products—had ostracized her from her family. With her earnings from sex work, she had built a small one-room house on her mother's land. Now, her stepfather had taken over the home in an attempt to kick her out. Finally, in this last fight, her stepfather had severely beaten her. Her mother accompanied her to the general hospital, told them she was there for substance abuse treatment, and left.

DR. TUN: It does look like she abandoned you at the hospital. Look, I have some information here. It says here you were admitted to the General Hospital due to substance abuse and were very worked up, and then they sent you here from there. You're right, nobody has been answering our calls, we've tried to reach your family, and nobody answers.

MARIBEL: I told my mother I want to be divorced from the two of them. I can't live like this.

DR. TUN: Divorced? You mean from your mother and stepfather?

MARIBEL: Yes. I don't want them in my life any more.

DR. TUN: So how can we help? What do you need from us?

MARIBEL: I want you to not leave me to fight this alone. I want to press charges against that man. I want to find my husband. I haven't seen him in eight, maybe ten years.

DR. TUN: Okay Maribel, for now, I can tell you that we are going to locate your family, because they abandoned you and they cannot do that. We will take care of your injuries, and we will help you with filing charges against him, if you so wish.

After the interview ended and Maribel went back to her room, Carolina read through her file and summarized: "Maribel has a history of substance abuse but when she's been back here she's denied using drugs and toxicology reports have come back negative. The drug tests have expired so we have to trust her word that she hasn't consumed any substances. She's been a sex worker, though now she claims to live off charity. She is homeless right now because her mother won't let her in the house. Her children are doing well in school, which is right across the street from them."

Dr. Tun pulled out a packet of *Galletas Marías*, a mild, sweet cracker very commonly eaten in Mexico, from her desk. She offered both of us a cracker and chewed thoughtfully and took the file back from Carolina. "Dr. Patrón admitted her," she said as she read through the file. "He says she is 'definitely psychotic.' But I don't see it. She's been here six times before and—ah!" she exclaimed, as she found the information she was looking for. "I treated her. I thought her case seemed familiar." She sighed. "This poor girl. I saw her back when I was in the long-term ward. If I were there," she continued, "I would have social work arrange a shelter to take her in. Her situation at home is untenable. But here, we are completely focused on acute care, so the social workers' goal is to locate the family and ensure they are involved. Maribel's problem is a lack of resources. She's illiterate, she has a small cognitive impairment, she's ignorant of her rights. She is very easy to take advantage of. This has happened before: she goes off and disappears for days, and while she is gone her mother and stepfather move in and take over the house and kick her out."

When Maribel's mother was finally located after a few days, she came to the hospital and met with Dr. Tun. Her version of events differed in intention, but not in substance: in fact, Maribel had disappeared for a few days. Concerned about Maribel's children, who are still minors, her mother and her husband moved in to look after them. A few days later, Maribel came back, filthy, intoxicated, and aggressive. A fight broke out. Her mother did not see how the situation could be improved without confining Maribel and getting her under control, so she took her to the hospital, informed the staff that Maribel was schizophrenic and on drugs, and left.

After that meeting, a frustrated Dr. Tun rubbed her temples, and sighed. As she and Carolina debriefed on the interview, Dr. Tun's frustration showed. "Maribel is suffering from schizophrenia," she remarked, "but her family, they can't see past the fact that she begs on the street and is a sex worker. To them, she isn't sick, she's a bad woman. And as long as we can't get them past that, it will be hard for us to help her. One thing is certain, though, this woman is not psychotic. She wasn't psychotic when she was brought in." Dr. Patrón had noted upon admission that she had appeared psychotic, but by the time she was evaluated by Dr. Tun, the symptoms had remitted, prompting Dr. Tun to conclude that Maribel had likely not been psychotic when she was admitted. It was possible that her temporary psychosis had been triggered by substances, as her mother claimed, but without testing strips, this was impossible to know.

LUCÍA

Lucía was committed to Las Lomas in mid-June 2012. When I came in to the office that morning, Dr. Tun and Carolina were holding the admissions clipboard, looking at it in dismay.

"Five admissions?" Dr. Tun said, shaking her head. This was an unusually high number.

"Why five?" Carolina speculated.

Dr. Tun examined the admissions roster and noted the names of the residents working that overnight shift. "Sometimes it's who has the overnight shift. Put certain doctors together, and they tend to admit more people than if they're alone or with others. At least we can send several people home today." She named several patients who were being sent home from the acute care ward, and those who were being moved to the long-term ward for further stabilization.

"Who do we have today?" I asked.

Carolina picked up the roster. "Lucía Robles," she read, "she's been here for two days. Yesterday she was too groggy for consultation. I'll go get her." She left the consultation room and Dr. Tun turned to me.

"This one is kind of interesting," she remarked, "Lucía thinks she is the governor of Yucatan. She was brought here under arrest for attacking some girls in her village, Tzucacab. I don't know much more than that, but let's see if we can find out."

A few minutes later, Carolina came back with a woman in her fifties. She was tall by Yucatecan standards, standing around five feet, seven inches. Her thick black hair framed her oval face like a lion's mane. She looked from Dr. Tun to me, then sat in the chair across Dr. Tun's desk.

"Good morning," Dr. Tun began the interview, "we met yesterday at your bed, but you were a little groggy. I'm glad to see you are doing better today. How did you sleep?"

"Fine," Lucía replied, "but I really need to be heading back to Tzucacab. We're about to change governments, and I can't be away right now."

DR. TUN: You mean because of the upcoming election?"

LUCÍA: That's right. If I'm not there, the monopolies come right in and take all of our support money. The free trade reforms, the structural adjustments, all of that, it's disrespectful. They took all the economic support. And I'm just asking for respect here. I'm the governor!

DR. TUN: You are the governor of where?

LUCÍA: Of here, of Yucatan.

DR. TUN: Isn't it Ivonne Ortega? Who is Ivonne Ortega if you are the governor?

LUCÍA: Look, what happens is this, I'm the one who pulls the strings. All of the collaborators throughout the different states, the funds are dispersed throughout all of the state government, the police, government, the municipal presidents. But when they saw the work I was doing they didn't like it, so they usurped my power, and this is why I don't like people making fun of me. And that girl, last week, I don't like her. If she has a problem with me, why doesn't she come talk to me? All she does is make fun of me behind my back, tell my son he doesn't have to obey me, making faces at me, laughing at me. And I am sorry, maybe I shouldn't have thrown rocks at her, but they were the ones to start it.

DR. TUN: You mean the children.

LUCÍA: Yes, the children. They taunt me and make fun of me. It's disrespectful! I'm the governor. I've been preparing this structural readjustment since I was a child, and this is how they repay me!

Lucía was, in many ways, a mystery. Her history revealed that she had been committed to Las Lomas eight times in her life. She had completed a high school education but had never left her home village. But we knew little else of her life history. I found her statements quite interesting because they were rife with neoliberal developmentalist discourse: she talked of "structural readjustments," "monopolies," and "free trade," though it was not clear that she knew what these terms meant. The conversation continued:

DR. TUN: Are you sick? Do you suffer from any illnesses?

LUCÍA: No, not at all. This is only the second time I come here.

DR. TUN: I think you've been here several times. Your file says you've been here about eight times.

LUCÍA: No, no, that's wrong.

DR. TUN: You don't remember being here?

LUCÍA: No, I'm telling you, that wasn't me. It wasn't me. It was someone else who pretended to be me. There's a woman who is wrong in the head and she comes in my name. You have to understand how they have worked against me, the horrible things they say. They say, "poor woman, she abandoned her children, she can't do anything."

DR. TUN: People say this about you?

LUCÍA: Yes, that's what people say about me. But they are all in the governor's web, this is all her doing.

DR. TUN: So there are two governors? You and someone else?

LUCÍA: That's what I'm coming to find out! But I'm telling you, I give orders, and they are followed. Whatever the governor does, I'm sending her the orders, like through, maybe telepathy. Or by fairy.

DR. TUN: What is this "fairy"?

LUCÍA: It's a system of government.

DR. TUN: That's its name? "Fairy"?

LUCÍA: I have a fairy for them.

DR. TUN: What is that, though? I have heard of fairies that have wings, like from the stories, is that what you mean?

LUCÍA: Yes, that's what I mean. See, I work through nature. I don't do any harm, I only do good. And you know what people did? Just pure evil, to suck me into their problems. I kept enacting these programs and they never funded them.

DR. TUN: Look, there is a document here that says you are here in custody. Your situation is that I cannot let you go until you are stable. I have to produce a document stating that your circumstances have changed, but they haven't yet, so I can't do it.

LUCÍA: But I can't stay! The change in political power is coming up, election day is July 2nd. And I have to go.

DR. TUN: So what should I do?

LUCÍA: Look, to begin with, a slap across the face isn't a crime. I am not in agreement with this. Bring me the governor, the police, someone who is trained, to sort this out. I was lied to! First they told me they were just taking me to Merida to get looked at by a doctor, and they brought me here. Then the doctor invited me to stay for two, maybe three days, and here you're telling me I'm in custody! I am not going to be stripped of my political office! I refuse. I did my job, I was a good governor. And what have I gotten? Mistreatment. Abuse. I disagree with this.

DR. TUN: You have to understand, my hands are tied . . .

LUCÍA: This is up to you, you do have the power! Why would they leave me here, if I'm not sick? What you all are doing is you're trying to keep all the funding, and I won't accept that from anyone from any political party.

Lucía became more and more agitated during the exchange as she realized that Dr. Tun was not going to release her. She tapped her index finger on the table for emphasis. As the conversation continued, Dr. Tun stopped trying to convince Lucía that she had no legal authority to release her from the hospital and instead tried to reassure her that she would likely return home before July 1, the date she believed the change in government was taking place. The election was two weeks away, she said comfortingly. Surely this would be resolved before then. Gradually, Lucía began to calm down, and she finally accepted Dr. Tun's reasoning that two weeks was plenty of time to resolve her situation and have her back in Tzucacab by election day. When Dr. Tun felt she had sufficiently de-escalated Lucía's state of mind, she sent her back to the ward.

Dr. Tun let out an exasperated laugh. "Goodness! That is a well-entrenched delusion!" she exclaimed as Carolina returned from escorting Lucía back to the ward.

CAROLINA: Sure, it's entrenched, but it's not very well structured. I mean, she says she's the governor, but she governs by fairy? Is she on any medication?

DR. TUN: She's isn't on anything. I think this poor girl is going to ECT [electroconvulsive therapy].

BEATRIZ: Why?

DR. TUN: Because she won't come out of it otherwise. Her delusion is too firm. I was going to show her the legal paperwork to explain why I couldn't release her, but I decided not to, I thought it would agitate her more.

CAROLINA: She settled down, she was fine when I walked her back to her bed.

DR. TUN: But as you say, her delirium isn't well-structured. She can't explain a lot of her ideas, they're confused. It's not systematic. She can't explain how or why she's governor. These are delusional ideas, but it's not a full-fledged delusion. But she does have delusional interpretations, delusional behavior.

Dr. Tun and Carolina believed, based on her file and interview, that Lucía had been arrested for hitting and throwing rocks at a child in Tzucacab. It was likely, according to Lucía's story, that the child had been part of a group who had been routinely making her life difficult through taunts and other kinds of abuse. Lucía had finally snapped, and the parents had decided to press charges against her. Given her extensive psychiatric history, Lucía had already lost custody of her own children, but Tzucacab was small enough that she still saw them frequently and still tried to mother them.

Dr. Tun, convinced that Lucía was not going to respond quickly enough to medication, scheduled her ECT after this meeting. ECT is a medical procedure whereby the patient, under general anesthesia, is administered a muscle relaxant, then is exposed to a series of electric shocks to the brain, triggering a seizure. ECT-induced seizures should last between 40–60 seconds. If a seizure lasts for longer than a minute, a rescue medication, usually a benzodiazepine, is used to stop it. At Las Lomas, ECT treatments generally took place over several days.

Prior to the emergence of pharmaceutical antipsychotics, ECT was frequently used as a form of treatment in psychiatric institutions throughout the world, but little is known about how ECT works to relieve psychiatric symptoms. Alongside psychosurgery (lobotomy), it became one of the most notorious symbols of psychiatric torture and abuse in the anti-psychiatry movement, as patients and advocates pointed to the long-term harms associated with its widespread use and propensity for abuse (Shorter and Healy 2012). Although it is no longer considered best practice in psychiatry, ECT has some demonstrated effectiveness as an antipsychotic (Correll et al. 2009; Tharyan and Adams 2003; Petrides et al. 2001). However, the reason it is considered a treatment of last resort is that, although effective, the treatment produces serious side effects, most notably in the form of short-term memory loss, and it can result in other serious brain damage in the long term. Because patients experiencing psychotic symptoms are incapable of providing informed consent for the procedure, in order to authorize the use of ECT, psychiatrists must obtain authorization from family members. If none are available to provide consent, a legal process must be undertaken, and the treatment must be authorized by a judge. With Lucía in custody and no family members in charge, it was legally easier to obtain authorization to move forward with the treatment than if she had had relatives involved in her care.

A few days later, Lucía's ECT treatment began. By her second treatment, her thinking had become, in Dr. Tun's words, "much more ordered and logical," though she still spoke of having political aspirations. She continued to insist she did not suffer from any illness. "Lucía would do extremely well if she only complied with her medication regimen," Dr. Tun lamented as she and Carolina debriefed after consultation, "but she doesn't believe she is sick, and her social environment doesn't help her at all." Dr. Tun decided that she would not release Lucía to the long-term ward, but instead opted to prescribe a monthly injectable antipsychotic once Lucía's psychosis fully remitted. This way, Lucía would be guaranteed to remain asymptomatic for a month, giving her time to come to terms with her condition. If she continued to comply with monthly injections, she would not have to take daily medication and would not sink back into yet another psychotic state. "As long as she doesn't accept that she's sick, though," Dr. Tun said, "she will probably not comply with her meds, and we will see her here again."

In this instance, Dr. Tun sees Lucía's inability to accept reality—that she is suffering from schizophrenia and that she needs to be continually medicated—as the most important obstacle to her recovery. Throughout their interactions, Dr. Tun tried to convince Lucía of this truth, although the excerpts I presented here show she also carefully navigates their conversations so as to avoid agitating her or reentrenching her delusion. Lucía's story reveals the existence of two regimes of truth: one in which Lucía is the fairy governor of Yucatan, manipulating nature to do her bidding, the other in which she is a seriously mentally ill woman, alone and vulnerable. The two regimes coexist, yet the former is subsumed into the latter, as Dr. Tun has the ultimate ability to obliterate the former through medical intervention.

DON GUSTAVO

As I describe in chapter 3, Dr. Patrón often used the psychiatric emergency room as a sort of outpatient clinic: rather than committing patients, he often would see patients in crisis, prescribe medication, and ask them to return in a week or two. Although patients were hospitalized at Las Lomas on a daily basis, many patients did not go through the emergency room, but rather were offered admission or committed during regular outpatient consultations. In my time observing Dr. Patrón, none of the patients visiting the emergency room during regular hours were committed. As I described in chapter 3, physician-patient consultations were usually attended by several people throughout the hospital's various departments, with the attending psychiatrist in charge (Dr. Patrón in the emergency room) and at least one resident. When I rotated into the emergency room, there were usually three, sometimes four, residents accompanying Dr. Patrón.

When Don Gustavo, who I introduced in chapter 4, came to the emergency room at Las Lomas accompanied by his wife, daughters, and granddaughter, all five of them came into the examination room. During his consultation, two residents, Ana and Daniela, were present. Don Gustavo, who had long been suffering from dementia, was going through a difficult time. As he and his wife sat down, and the remaining daughters and granddaughter stood behind their chairs, he looked at Dr. Patrón and sighed. *No tengo alivio*, "I have no relief," he said.

"He has no relief," his eldest daughter agreed, "he's worse right now than he was. He doesn't sleep. He walks around all night, banging on things. He fell. And we want to know where they can give him medication."

As I described in chapter 4, Don Gustavo's family had had a very difficult time procuring his medication even though Don Gustavo was an IMSS beneficiary. In their desperation, they had finally decided to seek help at Las Lomas. Dr. Patrón let his senior resident, Ana, take the lead on the interview:

ANA: How long has he been like this?

WIFE: It's been some two years that he's like this, although he goes through seasons when he gets better. I have been taking him to El Seguro for years, and they won't listen to us.

DANIELA: Is he aggressive?

DAUGHTER: Yes

DON GUSTAVO: No.

DAUGHTER: He has been suffering from this illness for two years, but now he's worse. I have seen how he gets aggressive. Yesterday he slapped my mother.

ANA: Where did you come from?

WIFE: Celestún.

DR. PATRÓN: Does he have schooling?

WIFE: A little.

DR. PATRÓN: Does he know how to read and write?

WIFE: A little.

DR. PATRÓN: How did the problem begin?

WIFE: He started seeing people, started saying he had found me with another man.

ANA: What date is today?

DON GUSTAVO: Tuesday.

ANA: What month?

DON GUSTAVO: I don't remember.

ANA: What year is this?

DON GUSTAVO: 1999.

ANA: Is it night time or day time right now?

DON GUSTAVO: It's day time, it's night time.

ANA: What do you mean?

WIFE: It's that he doesn't want to talk anymore.

DON GUSTAVO: No, day or night, it's the same.

DR. PATRÓN: How does he sleep?

[to his wife]

DON GUSTAVO: Very well, very well. That's one thing, I sleep very well.

WIFE: No, he doesn't sleep.

DR. PATRÓN: How does he eat?

[to his wife]

WIFE: He hasn't eaten since yesterday.

DON GUSTAVO: I eat just fine. What I don't like is having people talk about me without asking me directly.

GRANDDAUGHTER: The problem is IMSS. They prescribe medication but then IMSS doesn't have it in stock.

This interaction highlights the way that patients who come in to use Las Lomas's services must interact with many people, and the eclipsing effect that the involvement of multiple providers and family members can have on the experiences and desires of patients. The diagnostic event is one that involves residents developing expertise and patient families who ultimately have the power to make decisions over patient lives. As Ana tries to get a sense of Don Gustavo's orientation in time and space (*"Is it night time or day time right now?"*), Don Gustavo's wife speaks on his behalf to explain his answer (*"he doesn't want to talk anymore"*). Ana ignores her because he has given her the answer she is looking for: he is not oriented in time and space, a serious symptom of his worsening dementia.[6] At other points in the interview, Don Gustavo is completely ignored as he repeatedly attempts to answer for himself the questions that Dr. Patrón and the residents pose to his family members.

In this exchange, Ana, the resident, is trying to ascertain Don Gustavo's orientation. In a sense, she, too, is trying to orient herself both in relationship to Don Gustavo, whom she at first directs herself to, and with Don Gustavo's large family, who are actively participating in the interview. As we can see from the conversation transcript, Don Gustavo is oriented enough to know that he is being spoken about: "What I don't like," he says, "is having people talk about me." However, once Ana ascertains that he is not oriented in time and space, she stops interacting with him and begins interacting with his family. His annoyance goes unacknowledged by everyone in the room as the conversation continues without him. Without orientation, he cannot be a neoliberal, autonomous subject, and thus the conversation must continue with those who can make decisions on his behalf. The possibilities of negotiation are gone. Meanwhile, Dr. Patrón and his residents are also orienting themselves to the practical challenges faced by

Don Gustavo and his family, who are unable to access needed medication through the Seguro Social.

Don Gustavo's personhood is crushed under the overwhelming weight of the diagnostic process. As his responses reveal his disorientation in the world, his relatives and physicians zone him into nonbeing. By the same token, Ana's urging of Don Gustavo's family to enroll in Seguro Popular, and Dr. Patrón's tacit support of her proposal (described in detail in chapter 4), also reveal an active interest on the part of the physicians to avoid institutionalization. Ana sees the family struggling with the worsening challenge of caring for Don Gustavo, who is becoming aggressive and increasingly a danger to himself and others, and she tries to help them from within her own limited scope of action as an advanced psychiatric resident. Dr. Patrón, too, tries to help, simplifying Don Gustavo's medication regimen. However, as described in chapter 4, the difficulty of procuring the medication, much of which is still under patent and therefore prohibitively expensive, echoes Taussig's (1987) descriptions of medical care in Colombia, where sick and dying babies are prescribed tests and treatments their parents can never afford. At the heart of Ana's and Dr. Patrón's attempts to help this struggling family is an unspoken recognition that without family involvement and support Don Gustavo's options are nonexistent, particularly in a remote community like Celestún.

In the acute care ward, Dr. Pacheco, Dr. Castro, and Dr. Tun all hold positions in Mexico's greater medical community: all three are permanent, essentially tenured physicians in one of Mexico's public health care institutions. They enjoy job security, a regular salary, and the coveted pension benefits associated with employment in the state and federal government. All three are also engaged in some degree of pedagogy at local universities beyond the supervision of psychiatric and integrative medicine residents in the institution itself. Dr. Tun's position requires her to be engaged in research as well. In addition, all three maintain private practices. Dr. Pacheco, Dr. Castro, and Dr. Tun are successful psychiatrists, well respected by their peers.

When I first met Dr. Tun, she was actively involved in Dr. Vasquez's suicide prevention support group. Initially, she was the attending psychiatrist in Las Lomas's emergency room, the first line of assessment. Between 2008 and 2013, Dr. Tun was promoted from being in charge of the psychiatric emergency room to the position of attending psychiatrist of women in the psychiatric acute care ward after a brief stint in the long-term women's ward. Dr. Tun and I became friendly over years of ethnographic visits. Her interest in research and her respect for anthropological approaches—possibly related to the fact that Dr. Vasquez, an anthropologist by training, was her mentor—made her a valuable ally over the years, particularly during the time I spent in the acute care ward. I got to know her better than any of the other psychiatrists on the ward.

Dr. Tun was a bit of a renegade at Las Lomas. A psychoanalytic psychiatrist by training, she used medications sparingly in her own private practice, and frequently ran into trouble with Las Lomas's nursing staff, who at different points accused her of undermedicating her patients. Her psychoanalytic orientation also put her in the minority compared with most of her colleagues, who embraced bio-medical psychiatry. Born to a largely assimilated Yucatecan family with Maya heritage, Dr. Tun's history with Las Lomas went back to her years in medical school, when she moonlighted by working the overnight shift at Las Lomas to make extra money. Having studied with Dr. Vasquez, and then having worked for him at Las Lomas during his years directing the institution, Dr. Tun identified with his psychoanalytic approach and was an ally to him when I first arrived at Las Lomas in 2008. By 2012, Dr. Tun's own career was advancing and, though she remained on good terms with him, she was no longer a member of this inner cir-cle. Dr. Tun seemed to know how to navigate the difficult politics of Las Lomas: she was well-respected by her colleagues and got along with hospital administra-tors despite her occasional run-ins with the nursing staff.

By the time I began my work at Las Lomas in 2012, Dr. Tun was attending psy-chiatrist to the women in the acute care ward. In my official capacity as a researcher in the La Esperanza program, Dr. Tun generously welcomed me into her office, and later on she introduced me to the other two attending psychiatrists, who also allowed me to sit in as an observer on their consultations. Dr. Tun's patients were those who were either uninsured, their insurance status had not been verified, or they were covered by Seguro Popular—in other words, her patients— and Dr. Castro's—were indigent, low-income, or unemployed.

Dr. Castro is a slight man of medium build. In his youth, he spent his year of *servicio social*—a required year of social service following the completion of med-ical school—in a remote village in southern Yucatan. Dr. Castro does not speak Maya and stated his family has not spoken it for generations. He wears his jet-black hair slicked back and prefers a short-sleeved white *chaqueta*, a zippered, collared jacket, to the long-sleeved doctor's coat worn by Dr. Tun and Dr. Pacheco. As Las Lomas's acute care ward attending psychiatrists, Dr. Castro and Dr. Tun spend the most time in the ward. In contrast, Dr. Pacheco only visits the ward in the morning. This is because Las Lomas is only one part of Dr. Pacheco's work for IMSS; he spends the rest of his time providing psychiatric services in other IMSS institutions.

The shifts in the acute care ward worked in the following way: the attending psychiatrist was ultimately responsible for all the patients assigned to his or her care. However, rounds were conducted three times a day by psychiatry residents, who assessed patient process throughout the day and night. Residents were also charged with the overnight shift. Residents could prescribe medications and admit patients with a preliminary diagnosis, but they did not have the authority to diag-nose them once they were admitted or release them. As a teaching hospital, med-ical students and psychiatry and integrative medicine residents played an active role in the diagnosis and treatment of patients. Advanced residents in both the psychiatry and integrated medicine specialties were able to treat patients on their own in the hospital's outpatient services. These players—residents, students, nurses, cleaning staff, and social workers, plus doctors, patients, and family members—all navigated the spaces of the psychiatric hospital, a space that was at once open and suffocating, peaceful and tense, idyllic and horrific.

MARIANA

Dr. Tun also used negotiation as a strategy with her patients, but she sometimes resorted to confrontation as well. Mariana was a young woman who was committed by her mother.

DR. TUN: Why are you here?

MARIANA: Because of my mother, I guess. I don't like that her son-in-law is living in the house, like it's nothing. Spending time with my children, no, no, no, I don't agree with this. It's not like they have a large house, like we don't run into each other. That man should not be there.

DR. TUN: So how long have the problems been going on with him?

MARIANA: As far as I'm concerned, that man should not be there. He's just there, with his girlfriend, in my mother's house, like it's nothing!

DR. TUN: Okay, so how are you—I mean, when you leave here, I suppose you are going back there. How are you going to make sure you can coexist with him?

MARIANA: There is no coexisting with him. He shouldn't live there anymore. He fights with me. He hits me. He just shouldn't live there anymore.

DR. TUN: And what can you do? How are you going to solve this? When you are released, maybe on Saturday morning, are you going back to that house? To your house? The house your children live in? How are you going to get along with them?

MARIANA: It is impossible to coexist with that person.

DR. TUN: So how are you going to solve it?

MARIANA: You can scold her.

DR. TUN: I should scold your mother?

MARIANA: Yes. Tell her it's wrong for that man to live there.

In this instance, Dr. Tun's strategy has failed. Dr. Tun attempts to get Mariana to recognize that she is going to have to find a way to coexist with her antagonist by directly asking her, *How will you solve this?* But Mariana doesn't take the bait: by responding with *there is no coexisting with him*, she rejects Dr. Tun's very premise that Mariana has to coexist with her antagonist. Dr. Tun tries again. *But how are you going to solve this?* And again, Mariana replies, *it is impossible to coexist with this person.* The third—and final—time that Dr. Tun asks Mariana how she is planning on dealing with the situation, Mariana offers an unacceptable solution: *you scold her.*

To understand the inherent unacceptability of Mariana's offer, it is important to make note of the word she uses. Mariana uses is the Spanish *regañar* (scolding). *Regañar* is what parents do to misbehaving children. It goes against the patient empowerment rhetoric of twenty-first-century Mexican medicine. Scolding is not what doctors working in a twenty-first-century hospital should do to their patients or to patient families, yet medical scolding has been identified as a common contemporary problem in Latin American medical practice (Simpson 1988; Smith-Oka 2013; Lucas d'Oliveira et al. 2002). By using this word, Mariana is refusing to allow Dr. Tun to relinquish her authority—at the same time that she refuses Dr. Tun's attempts to lead her to a goal that can be actualized. The truth Dr. Tun was trying to negotiate was that Mariana could find a way to coexist with others in her household. Mariana, however, refused to do what Manuela did: she refused to acknowledge that her story had to change. The consequence of this refusal to negotiate the truth was that her record would fail to show the necessary progress to get her released.

FINDING ONE'S WAY IN THE OUTPATIENT CLINIC

Most patients who use Las Lomas's services do so on an outpatient basis. Las Lomas is the only inpatient psychiatric facility in the region, although the other health care organizations, IMSS and ISSSTE, do provide outpatient psychiatric services. Thus, the majority of people who use Las Lomas's outpatient services are enrolled in Seguro Popular and became outpatients either through diagnosis in the emergency room or because of an inpatient stay. Patients who receive outpatient treatment generally meet with their psychiatrist on a monthly, bimonthly, or trimonthly basis—these meetings become less frequent as patients become more stable (psychiatrists recognize the difficulties imposed on patients and their families in making the trip to Merida, which can mean a significant hardship).

DR. TREVIÑO: Don't take more medication than what is prescribed, okay? Just one, every night. Did you come alone?
PATIENT: No, I came with my younger brother.
DR. TREVIÑO: Where do you live?
PATIENT: In Kinil.
DR. TREVIÑO: What is that, about two hours away from here?
PATIENT: Yes.
DR. TREVIÑO: Well, then I'm going to give you enough medication for two months. [As an aside, to me] This patient has paranoid schizophrenia, and like I told you, yesterday we didn't have the medication, but today we do.

Generally, regular appointments take place in the hospital's outpatient consultation rooms, which are assigned to specific psychiatrists. Psychiatry residents are also expected to do a rotation in this area during their training, so patients are also likely to have at least one extra person observing their appointment. Advanced residents will also have the opportunity to treat outpatients on their own. Dr. Treviño is not always eager to prescribe several months' worth of medication, particularly to people who are local, because Las Lomas is not immune to medication shortages.

A patient using Las Lomas's outpatient services will receive an appointment for a certain time of day on a specific date. The patient will probably try to arrive at Las Lomas well before her scheduled time, as she is likely to be scheduled with other patients to the same time slot, and patients are seen in the order that they arrive. Once she checks in, her file will be stacked in order with those of the other patients scheduled. The stack will then be walked to the doctor's office, and they will be placed on his desk. The patients then sit in the hallway and wait for their names to be called out. If the doctor arrives late, and consultations start late, then a patient with a 9 A.M. appointment may not actually see the doctor until 11 A.M. or later. This is not specific to Las Lomas, but it is a common practice in all Mexican health care and, as discussed in chapter 4, is typical of health services in resource-poor settings worldwide.

Dr. Treviño was well past the age of retirement. He clearly continued to do the work because he enjoyed it and had worked in some fashion at Las Lomas from the time it opened in 1970, and he had worked at its predecessor-institution before that. He was a mentor to my friend Juan and had worked under him as hospital subdirector in the 1980s and 1990s. In contrast to Dr. Tun, Dr. Treviño, even though he was a Frommian-trained psychoanalytic psychiatrist, did not shy away from a heavy reliance on pharmaceuticals to treat his patients, most of whom were diagnosed with schizophrenia. Like regular visits with psychiatrists in other parts of the world, Dr. Treviño's visits were generally short and consisted of a series of questions about recent symptoms, medication compliance, and recent life events. As was the case in consultations in the psychiatric emergency room, family members very often played an important part in the consulations in Dr. Treviño's office. In the following conversation, Doña Laura, a woman in late middle age, accompanied by her grown son, pays Dr. Treviño a medication visit. After a brief exchange of pleasantries, the following exchange occurs.

DR. TREVIÑO: How is she doing?
[to the patient's son]
SON: She still talks to herself, but just a little. She's been hiding, but just for short whiles.
LAURA: I just hear the voices.
DR. TREVIÑO: What do the voices say?
SON: She says they're annoying her.
DR. TREVIÑO: Do they use profanities? [trying to determine if the voices are persecutory]
SON: Yes

DR. TREVIÑO: So she is still hearing voices. Do you make sure she swallows the
   medicine?
SON: Yes, she swallows it.
LAURA: Yes, I take my medication.
DR. TREVIÑO: Is anyone trying to hurt you?
LAURA: Yes, he wants to hurt me.
DR. TREVIÑO: The man.
SON: But you don't live with him anymore, Mami, you live with me.
DR. TREVIÑO: She just identified her aggressor. It's his voice she's hearing, you
   know. But the medication she's taking, the Olanzepine, it's pretty strong, it should
   take the voices away.

Most of this exchange could well have taken place between Dr. Treviño and
Doña Laura's son. Her presence at first glance appears to be cursory. Doña Laura
attempts to speak for herself when Dr. Treviño asks her son if he is making sure
that she swallows her medication. Dr. Treviño's largely positive view on biomedical psychiatry shines through in the way he says, confidently, that the medication
is strong and should *take the voices away.*[7]

Las Lomas provides psychiatric services to over 60,000 patients a year, most
of whom use its outpatient services. Thus, even though patients are assigned a single psychiatrist with the idea of providing a continuity of care, regular visits can
often appear to be no different than first visits. In the following example, the
patient, Georgina, had been using Las Lomas's services off and on for the last four
years. When she and her mother arrived in Dr. Treviño's office, however, there
was some confusion. Carolina was assisting.

DR. TREVIÑO: Have a seat. Is this your mother?
GEORGINA: Yes
DR. TREVIÑO: Have a seat. How are you?
GEORGINA: Good

Dr. Treviño went through her case file, trying to figure out her medication regimen. He continued to review the case file for a few minutes, muttering different
medication names under his breath.

DR. TREVIÑO: The note on the file doesn't say much, or the handwriting is hard to
   make out.

He showed it to Carolina. As she reviewed the file, a nurse came in with another
stack of patient files and placed them on his desk. It became clear that this was
Georgina's first time visiting Dr. Treviño. What was not clear was Georgina's
history.

CAROLINA: She was committed in August of 2009 for six days. Diagnosed with depressive disorder with psychotic symptoms and suicidal ideation. She was released of her own accord. She came back for follow-up treatment in outpatient. She explained that she had been feeling sadness for the last three months, crying, hearing voices. She could sleep, but she felt the sleep wasn't restful. One day, she had to leave her work because of a crying fit.

GEORGINA: I have a new job now. I've been working for four months without incident.

As Carolina tried to make sense of the garbled handwriting in Georgina's file, Dr. Treviño observed Georgina's demeanor. As he observed her, he began to make his assessment, speaking about her to Carolina before asking Georgina if she had suicidal ideation at the moment.

DR. TREVIÑO: Well, today she seems properly oriented in time, space, and person. Her affect and language are coherent and competent. You seem to be doing well, do you have any suicidal ideas?

GEORGINA: No.

DR. TREVIÑO: Any delirium? Seeing things that aren't there?

CAROLINA: This says you saw shadows that said your name?

GEORGINA: That's right.

At this point, Carolina and Dr. Treviño were conducting the assessment together. However, as Dr. Treviño further questioned Georgina, Carolina's role changed, and she fell into the background, taking notes.

DR. TREVIÑO: Shadows? What were they like?

GEORGINA: The shadows? I couldn't tell you.

DR. TREVIÑO: What did the shadow belong to? A man or a—

GEORGINA: A person, a man.

DR. TREVIÑO: And did it say things?

GEORGINA: No. I just see them pass.

DR. TREVIÑO: And are you semi-asleep, almost asleep when you see them?

GEORGINA: No.

DR. TREVIÑO: Is it when you are awake?

GEORGINA: Yes, when I am awake.

DR. TREVIÑO: Could you be mistaken? Could it be you just thought you saw something? Could it be your fear?

GEORGINA: I think so, because I get scared when I'm left alone at home.

DR. TREVIÑO: It could be your fear, or could it be that someone was in your house? Listen, tell me the truth, what you think.

GEORGINA: What I think. . . .

DR. TREVIÑO: If you really believe that there was someone there who wanted to harm you, and you feel that and think it, you say so.

GEORGINA: Uh-huh . . .

DR. TREVIÑO: I'm not going to try to convince you. I just want to know exactly what you think [chuckle] that gives me a better orientation. Hmm? Knowing what you think.

GEORGINA: Maybe it's my fear of being left alone at home.

DR. TREVIÑO: "Maybe," you say? "Maybe."

GEORGINA: Yes.

DR. TREVIÑO: You have some doubt. But back then, in that moment, you thought someone was trying to harm you.

Dr. Treviño's questions were purposeful, but also hurried. He did not give Georgina time to think over her answers—what do the shadows look like? Do they speak? He did not contradict or question the fact that she denied the shadows speak but said they spoke in the past. However, the fact that he exhorted her to *tell the truth* suggests he doubted her. At the same time, Georgina herself seemed unsure. She replied by repeating the question—*what I think*—or by acknowledging the question without answering it—*uh-huh*. At one point, perhaps sensing that Georgina was unsure of how to answer, Dr. Treviño took a moment to explain. *I'm not trying to convince you*, he said, of whether there was someone in Georgina's house trying to harm her. *I want to know exactly what you think*, he said, and then he chuckled at the idea. When Georgina finally said, *maybe*, Dr. Treviño concluded that Georgina was properly oriented in time and space—and therefore, not paranoid. If she had doubt, and she did not have doubt before, then she was not delusional. At the same time, Dr. Treviño's questioning itself introduced doubt. He asked, *Could you be mistaken?*

PATIENT: Yes. I think I was very *alterada*, with many nights without sleep. It was too much, and the things I was seeing, I took them seriously.

DR. TREVIÑO: It says here she had suicidal ideation at one point?

CAROLINA: Yes, her prior—the first time that she was admitted.

DR. TREVIÑO: You remember that, right?

GEORGINA: Yes.

DR. TREVIÑO: Why did you want to kill yourself?

GEORGINA: Because I had a lot of things that came into my head. Problems.

DR. TREVIÑO: What kinds of things came into your head?

GEORGINA: Sometimes when my parents fought. Or when I fought with my parents.

DR. TREVIÑO: When you had disagreements with your parents.

GEORGINA: Uh-huh. They would tell me something I did wrong, and I didn't like that. Problems with my siblings, when they said things to me.

DR. TREVIÑO: And what kinds of things could they tell you? Were they so bad?

GEORGINA: Uh-huh. You get into fights with them, or they don't like something, they get upset. Things like that. Things would come into my mind. . . .

DR. TREVIÑO: Huh. Did it appear at some point that she had schizo? And then at another that it was depression?

CAROLINA: Depression. Major depression with psychotic symptoms.

DR. TREVIÑO: At admission?

CAROLINA: At admission.

DR. TREVIÑO: I would add a question mark to that. [To patient] Were you seeing things? Hearing things?

GEORGINA: At that time, yes.

DR. TREVIÑO: And you thought they were against you?

GEORGINA: Hmmmmmm, yes.

DR. TREVIÑO: And they wanted to harm you?

GEORGINA: Yes.

DR. TREVIÑO: Was that what was making you sad and making you cry? Was that bothering you? Tell me the truth. Or was it the problems with your brothers? Or was it all together? Only you can know that, only you can tell me.

GEORGINA: It was everything together that contributed to what happened to me. Because I heard the voices, I saw the things, any little thing altered me, made me nervous, I couldn't understand why.

Again, Dr. Treviño exhorted Georgina to *tell the truth*. But he also made it very clear to Georgina what he expected the truth to be, and that he needed her to make that claim. What is the truth? What does it mean to arrive at mutually agreed upon truth through a process of negotiation that is largely based on the patient and physician's ability to orient themselves toward one another? Psychiatric patients are uniquely vulnerable; their freedom is at the mercy of doctors who decide whether they are rational enough to function as productive, self-actualizing neoliberal subjects.

Dr. Patrón's exchange with Manuela demonstrates that the inherent "trueness" of the patients' words is not nearly as important as their believability. Dr. Treviño recognizes that "the truth" is something only the patient can know; yet he guides her—no, he *orients her*—toward the particular truth he needs her to articulate. Truth in this instance is enthroned in negotiation as well as violence (Rose 1996, 55) because if the truth offered is not satisfying, the doctor has the ability take the patient's freedom. The actual truth—the "really real," if there is such a thing— is irrelevant. Some rationality is a prerequisite to this negotiation. Don Gustavo, unable to prove he is oriented enough to be rational, loses his ability to arrive at his own negotiated truth. Manuela, incoherent and lost for the first month of her internment, was confined in isolation. Mariana, in contrast, drives a hard bargain because she refuses to concede in her negotiation.

In these pages, I have demonstrated how truth, negotiation, and orientation operate in the interactions between doctors and patients. It quickly becomes apparent that, for the doctors and the patients in the wards, the "truth" is far from self-evident: it is a negotiated arrangement at the heart of which are human beings seeking to orient themselves toward one another. The truth is enshrined in violence because the arbiter of negotiation is the doctor who decides whether the patient is a person to be released or a body to be managed. Moreover, each of these psychiatric encounters reveals the inner workings and reproduction of the colonial matrix of power; rather than being a simple unidirectional system of oppression, it becomes clear that social interactions and relationships weave together in an intricate web of social relations. In chapter 6, I describe what this means in the heart of madness: the subjective experience of psychosis.

6 · IN THE HEART OF MADNESS

> The only part I could ever understand was a riddle about loss and emergence
> and it went like this: Why are you here if you cannot put yourself in my
> place?　　　　　　　　　　　　　—Lucas Bessire, *Behold the Black Caiman*

WEARING THE WHITE COAT

Ethnographic fieldwork in a psychiatric institution can be challenging work. As I
discussed in chapter 1, a primary concern throughout this process was to ensure
that the work was carried out in an ethical manner. Almost immediately, I encountered a conundrum. Dr. Tun always introduced me as "Beatriz, the anthropologist" to doctors and patients in the ward, to avoid confusion of using "doctor" in
the title. At the same time, from my first day in the acute ward, she took an extra
doctor's coat hanging on a hook in her office and handed it to me. I should always
wear the coat on the ward, she said. The paradox was somewhat striking to me:
the white coat clearly "marked" me—maybe not as a doctor, but as a nonpatient,
non-nurse, nonstaff, nonoutsider. The coat made me look like I belonged with the
doctors, even though I was "Beatriz, the anthropologist" and so *not* a medical doctor. The coat made it easy to move around the hospital, although I never ven-
tured into the locked wards by myself, and I was once stopped and questioned
by a suspicious nurse. The coat got me through security, and it anonymized me
to the other doctors and residents.

I experienced a profoundly disquieting feeling by donning the white coat. I had
full approval to be at Las Lomas as a member of Dr. Vasquez's team. Las Lomas's
administration knew about my presence, and my research had gone through IRB
screening at my institution, though I had not been required to go through additional review on site. Yet, the white coat made me uncomfortable. It felt as though
it was defining me to others before I could define or explain myself. And I wor-
ried that the coat might mislead the patients into thinking I was a medical professional, when I was not. But Dr. Tun's reasoning when I asked her why I should
wear it was implacable: "These are highly acute patients who are already confused
about where they are and who we are. Many of them are psychotic. Many of them
are paranoid. All of them are in crisis. The coat avoids adding more confusion."

Though she never explicitly said it, it was clear to me that in her role as attending psychiatrist and as my primary collaborator, she called the shots. So, I wore the coat.

The reader may wonder about the point of this story about the coat, my ambivalence, and what it did for me in my work at Las Lomas. In this instance, my point is this: when I don the white coat, it affects people and spaces around me in ways I cannot control. And I experience an ambivalent relationship with it. One could argue that the coat is imbued with the magic of the modern (Taussig 1987, 274), contaminating me with its ideologies, belief systems, and potentials. In 1980s Puerto Tejada, Colombia, Taussig describes shamanic healers who wear white coats and become possessed by the spirit of Colombian surgeon José Gregorio (281). In this possessed state, healers perform surgery and cure patients. On another level, the magic modern also describes the faith people have in doctors and biomedicine even though the actual care they often receive from doctors who—in a practice evocative of the experiences faced by Don Gustavo and his family—request tests and prescribe medicines that their patients cannot ever afford, does very little to help them. When Dr. Tun asks me to wear the coat, I felt I was being asked to don some of its modern magic, to represent myself as part of this system. As a researcher, I was already a representative of another, also modern, and also colonial, system. The coat, in this sense, outed me as another modern colonial settler.

Years later, when I see pictures of myself wearing the white coat, my mixed feelings toward it reemerge. My concern about its effect on my relationship with the patients I interviewed returns along with happy memories of friendships formed and insight gained during my time at Las Lomas. What is interesting about the white coat is that it is at once material and relational. It is a physical object that absorbs me, the outside researcher, into the colonial matrix of power represented by the psychiatric institution. In *The Gender of the Gift* (1990), Marilyn Strathern argues that objects are repositories of relationships.[1] A materialist take on this argument might go one step further and say that the agency of objects lies in their inherent relationality. The coat, in the sense that it affects my relationships with all my interlocutors—patients, hospital staff, doctors—has agency.

The argument that objects have agency has been made before (Latour 2007; Bennett 2010), and this argument has been extended to engage with Invisible Beings as the objects of modern psychiatry and psychology (Latour 2013; Reyes-Foster 2016b). As described by Latour, Invisible Beings[2] are seen in traditional societies as the cause of symptoms "Moderns" consider psychiatric (Latour 2013, 181). However, as Latour and other anthropologists writing within the "ontological turn" have argued, it is one thing to apply a modern explanation to an ethnomedical (and therefore, nonmodern) etiology and quite another to take this etiology seriously (Viveiros de Castro 2014). In other words, Latour invites us to grant these Invisible Beings ontological status. In writing a new metaphysics, anthropologists writing in the ontological turn propose something that is interesting and innovative. By the same token, these metaphysical questions can quickly move toward the esoteric and away from the production of disparities, inequality, and social suffering on the ground.[3]

Nevertheless, the notion of exploring Invisible Beings from a perspective that grants them ontological status holds some promise. The acute ward is full of Others—Other Beings, Other Realities, Other Truths—with whom patients experience profound relationships. It is the primary responsibility of the psychiatrist to make these Others go away: the delusions, hallucinations and delirium must remit if "improvement" is to be measured. And yet, through my conversations with patients in the acute ward and my observations of their interactions with their attending psychiatrists, I soon found that the relationships between patients and their Others warranted further examination. That exploration of psychosis, what some might consider the heart of madness, may reveal something about the ways human beings—sane and mad—exist in the world in the context of the colonial matrix of power.

In this chapter, I explore the experiences of several psychiatric patients living in the heart of madness. Initially, this analysis will focus on the ways in which clothing and relationality coalesce, building on other anthropological, indigenous, and decolonial approaches to argue for an understanding of existence that is simultaneously material—in the sense of that which holds a tangible existence in the world—and relational—in connection with human and nonhuman agents that coexist in registers of visibility. These registers exist with asymmetrical and disparate abilities: while from a political economic perspective it may seem that helpless patients interact with powerful doctors who have the ability to decide over their immediate futures, this view moves beyond this paradigm, engaging with actors who are seldom visible in political-economic narratives but nevertheless have profound effects on everyone in the ward. Although the analysis begins with clothing, it soon expands to other visible and invisible actors in the context of coloniality, indigenous scholarship, and the so-called ontological turn in anthropology. As I have argued throughout this book, coloniality is not a zero-sum game or a unidirectional system of oppression, but a complex web of social processes constituted through the actions and interactions of actors on the ground. In this case, the actors in question are not merely the individual patients involved, or their doctors, but the beings that inhabit their own realities. By engaging in their stories, I explore the ways in which these people navigate their worlds in their everyday struggles.

"IN MY PROPER CLOTHING"

Clothing is important in Yucatecan society, as it is in many other places. It marks ethnicity, gender, and social class. In the psychiatric ward, it takes on new meaning. "You have to talk to Efrain," Dr. Castro, the men's attending psychiatrist, said to me, with some excitement in his voice, on a Monday morning in July 2012. "His case is fascinating, and he's moving wards today. I'll arrange for you to have a visit with him."

Thus I began to collect interviews in the acute care ward at Las Lomas in the summer of 2012. After I conducted participant observation research inside the wards for just over a month, the attending psychiatrists agreed that some of their patients who were capable of giving informed consent could be invited to participate in an interview. Efrain was the first patient I interviewed. Efrain smiled easily and nodded agreeably as I read the IRB-approved consent document I had prepared in Orlando.

"We can stop the interview at any time," I explained as he read through the standardized language of the consent document, "you do not have to participate in this interview if you don't want to. It's important to me that you don't feel like anyone is forcing you to talk me. . . ." I continued to verbalize the stipulations listed in the study consent document.

When I finished, Efrain nodded amiably and said he understood. We sat at a small plastic table on plastic chairs in the entrance of the acute care ward, an area that functions both as a dining hall and space for visitors to meet with their loved ones. The recording, made on my iPad as I typed out notes, picks up on the sounds of clattering plates and cups, and the clicking of my fingers on the keyboard. When I listened back to the interview as I wrote this chapter, I remembered that we talked just after visiting hours had ended, at noon, as the staff began setting up for lunch. Efrain and I talked about how he was feeling and how he felt he was treated by hospital doctors and staff. The interview was convivial, and it quickly took on the feel of conversation. Efrain smiled pleasantly and answered my questions thoughtfully and thoroughly.

The first question I asked him was "tell me about your experience here at the hospital." He explained that he had been very afraid of being hospitalized because he had been traumatized as a small child when he had had surgery. As we talked, though, Efrain emphasized his own sense of improvement—he had slept soundly the night before, he said, and had woken up at the time he usually woke up to go to work. He was anxious to get back to work.

EFRAIN: I even want to dress well already.
BEATRIZ: You don't like the uniform?
EFRAIN: I don't like it.
BEATRIZ: Why don't you like it?
EFRAIN: When I see myself, I don't like it. I feel like a sick person. I feel, I feel like . . .
    I feel sick. If I dressed in my proper clothing, I would be better.

Efrain's statement had caught my attention. He said the uniform made him feel like a sick person. It made him feel sick. I found this interesting, so I pursued this.

BEATRIZ: And do you think you are sick?
EFRAIN: No [he starts laughing].

Thus, though the uniform made him feel sick, Efrain knew was not sick—the idea was so ludicrous he laughed out loud.

BEATRIZ: Well, tell me, what is a sick person?
EFRAIN: [sighs] A sick person doesn't think about things carefully. He says things, or if not, he cries over any little thing, or if not, he can't walk because he's sick. All the time, he feels sad, that is a sick person, or he feels, like, an ogre, that is a sick person.

Efrain's definition of a sick person was directly the opposite of his own behavior. This was no coincidence. When I asked him to describe a healthy person, Efrain's description was that of a primarily agreeable person—someone who smiles, who is pleasant, who converses easily with others. Efrain was performing his own state of health for hospital staff—perhaps even including me—so that he could prove that he was not a sick person and therefore did not need to be at Las Lomas.

The power of the hospital patient's uniform—a green or blue cotton shirt and synthetic-blend shorts for the men and a shapeless blue or green cotton nightgown for the women—to affect Efrain's sense of self is evident in the way he talks about his experience as a patient inside the acute ward. In his words, the uniform could transform him from a healthy person into a sick one—or at least, it could make him *feel* sick. In the same way the white coat is imbued with the magic of the modern, so is the uniform. It contains the transformative power of biomedical illness categories, marking Efrain as a sick person even when he does not believe he is ill. Efrain's only recourse is performance: he will wear the uniform but act as if he were healthy.

Clothing plays an important role outside of Las Lomas as well. Its transformative potential is exemplified in Candy's story. As I sat across the table from Candy, I saw a thirty-eight-year-old woman with thick, curly black hair, wearing the women's hospital gown. She looked back at me with an expression that was simultaneously curious and suspicious. I introduced myself, explained that I was an anthropologist researching the experiences of patients at Las Lomas, and I asked if she would be willing to chat with me and answer a few questions. Candy explained that she had been committed because she had been "going around town telling people she was a boy." Candy's diagnosis was F44.7, "Conversion Disorder with mixed symptom presentation." Conversion disorder is classified by the ICD-10 (and the DSM-5) alongside dissociative disorders. It is a new name for one of the oldest and certainly the most famous disorder in psychiatric history: hysteria. At Las Lomas, this diagnosis seems to be made when psychiatrists cannot

quite fit the patient symptomology with any other diagnosis. Candy had been hospitalized when she had begun dressing and acting like a man, giving herself the
name "Anthony."

BEATRIZ: So what happened that made them bring you here?
CANDY: A boy and a girl passed.
BEATRIZ: A boy and a girl passed?
CANDY: Yes. Through me. I'm a girl, I'm a boy. I don't want to be a woman, nor a girl.
I want to be a man so that I can protect myself so that I'm not grabbed, or touched.
As a girl, I was abused by many people.
BEATRIZ: And this is why you were committed?
CANDY: Yes. Because I'm telling people that I'm Anthony. Anthony is a man. And
Lupita is a woman.

Candy explained that she never believed she was a man, but she had chosen to
dress and act like one. It was not that she wanted to be a man; rather, she did not
want to be a woman.

BEATRIZ: So you say you want to be a man?
CANDY: A boy.
BEATRIZ: Not a man, a boy.
CANDY: So that I am not touched. I dress like a man. I like it, but it's not because I
want to be a man, it's because I don't want to be a woman. I don't want to be
touched.
BEATRIZ: You don't want to be a woman.
CANDY: No. Because I have been touched by many. I have been mistreated. From the
time I was a child, when I was four years old I was abused, then when I was twelve,
I think, and then when was fifteen.
BEATRIZ: So girls are abused, but boys are not, so it is better to be a boy. What about
Lupita, then?
CANDY: Her too.
BEATRIZ: But Lupita is a woman.
CANDY: That one almost never comes out. Only Anthony comes out.
BEATRIZ: When was the last time Anthony came out? Has he come out since you've
been here?
CANDY: Fifteen days ago. But not right now. He won't come out now. . . . He comes
out when there is fighting.

Although she had initially told me that she was committed because of both
Anthony and Lupita, she stated later on that Lupita "almost never" came out.
Lupita was an innocent little girl, she explained—perhaps an idealized represen-
tation of the abuse-free girlhood Candy would have liked for herself. Candy did

not elaborate; she simply said the little girl was named Lupita because she wanted to be happy. When it came to Anthony, Candy had more to say. She explained that she had been involved in a stressful love triangle at the time that "the boy" manifested.

CANDY: I don't want them to fight among themselves, so that's why that boy came out, I think, a boy came out to defend [me], so that they wouldn't hurt each other.
BEATRIZ: So until that moment, the boy had never come out before, ever.
CANDY: No. But I did want to dress like a man.
BEATRIZ: I see.
CANDY: But I do it to protect myself, like I told you.
BEATRIZ: So the boy is protecting you.
CANDY: Yes. Because I dress like a boy. Big, wide clothes. Like a, like a *cholo*. That's how dress. I put on my baseball cap, my shoes, sneakers.
BEATRIZ: And how do you like to be called?
CANDY: Anthony.

Candy began donning male clothing well before she adopted Anthony's persona. Anthony protected her from conflict and abuse. The particular guise of masculinity she adopted, the cholo, is that of a quintessential "tough guy." When she becomes Anthony, one could argue she takes on the strengths of the cholo while assuaging the danger of an adult male by making him a male child.

For Efrain, clothing makes him feel as though he were an *enfermo*, a sick person, an identity category he rejects. For Candy, clothing functions to empower and protect her. Both ascribe transformative powers to clothes, yet both recognize that the transformation occurs in only one sense. Yes, clothes make Efrain feel like an enfermo, but he knows he really is not. Yes, clothes make Candy feel like a boy, momentarily taking away the female gender she wants to reject. But she also acknowledges she does not really turn into a boy when she is dressed as one, nor does she want it to. "I don't want to be a man," Candy says, "I just don't want to be a woman." At this juncture it is tempting to conjure Butler's performativity of gender; certainly, there is potential for that. However, I am more interested in the intersections of subjectivity and materiality—the way in which the vibrant materiality (Bennett 2010) of these objects reacts and is reacted upon by subject-patients. As Candy's story illustrates, these intersections are clearly gendered.

If objects have agency, vibrant materiality is one way of conceptualizing how this agency acts upon other things and beings. Vibrant materiality thus runs through and across human and nonhuman bodies. Another patient, Claudina, who I met in 2008, was committed to Las Lomas following a suicide attempt during a psychotic break. One day, as we were in a group therapy session for La

Esperanza, Dr. Vasquez's suicide prevention program, Claudina teared up as she explained a recent heartbreak:

> I grew up in a very humble home. And when I say humble, I don't mean that I only ate tortillas and beans, or that I only ate tomato and chile like my grandmother does. But with [my boyfriend], I started to see new things. I saw people that go into Costco. People that go into Walmart. . . . And this made me sad (her voice breaks) You know why? Because I cannot go to those places. I can only go look at the things they have, but I cannot buy anything. I'm used to buying second-hand clothes. My underwear, I buy it at the *tianguis*, and I wear it. I'm not ashamed to say it because I am used to poverty. . . . [My boyfriend] made fun of me because I wanted to read Moby Dick by Herman Melville. He said I was not going to understand it. But when I read it I found that Melville used a language that was not exactly difficult. It was explicit. It was elegant. I am always drawn to things which are elegant. But there is an elegance that comes from being a professional, and another that comes from mestizaje. My grandmother is a great wise woman, who has always taught me how things should be done in order to do them well.[4]

Claudina's discourse is rife with vibrant matter: the underwear she must buy at the *tianguis* (second-hand clothes market), *Moby Dick*, even her physical wounds. Each of these objects carries a transformative force that affects her existence. She uses her experience of buying second-hand clothing to illustrate her painful nature of poverty, which she contrasts to her grandmother's poverty, which is characterized by foods associated with a traditional diet. The fact that she has to explain that she is not ashamed to admit that her underwear comes from a tianguis betrays her awareness that others may see this as shame-worthy. It is interesting that Claudina spoke of her suicide attempt as a transformative experience and ascribed an external agency to her wounds even when she herself had created them. This exterior locus of agency, even one inscribed on the body itself, is not unlike the vibrant materialism of the uniform Efrain described in the interview I conducted four years later.

Claudina became an important person in my work at Las Lomas in 2008. On the second day after I met her, as she listened to others share their stories of hurt and strife that brought them to the edge of life,[5] she pointed to the ways in which she had hurt her body and concluded, "Our body is a temple of God, so we must adore our wounds, because they teach us what we shouldn't do." Claudina gave my dissertation a title.[6]

For Claudina, every wound on her body and that of others was a lesson tied to her own spirituality. These self-inflicted wounds carried the ability to transform her. The culmination of this transformation came in the form of the near-death experience she described after she attempted to hang herself: "I tried to kill myself, and then I had an extrasensory experience . . . words came to my mind, and those things made me hang myself. The voices told me life wasn't worth it, that I should kill myself. I started to look for God, and I saw a little light, which became a white light with black spots. But God didn't choose to take me. He gave me a new life."

Ontology attempts to understand the nature of existence. Mol (2003) argues that there no single ontology to be taken for granted. Things do not exist in and of themselves but are, rather, brought into being in daily sociomaterial practice (6). This framework allows us to think of everyday existence as inherently socio-material: that is, social interactions mediate, interact with, or include material objects. In each instance outlined so far here, we can subtextually infer multiple ontologies brought into being by the sociomaterial practices that bind clothing, lights, and scars. There are other vibrant materials that patients in the psychiatric ward must interact with: food, medications, ligatures, walls, locks, toilets. For the patients, these materials are a source of horror and distress. However, materiality may be limiting with its focus on the material. What about nonhuman actors that are immaterial, but real to the people in the ward?

While the works of new materialisms scholars like Coole and Frost (2010) and Bennett (2010) encourage us to see materials as "productive, not simply static, dead, acted upon" (TallBear 2016, 10), Kim TallBear (2016) observes that the "New Materialisms" are not so new. As TallBear points out, "The new materialists may take the intellectual intervention that grounds the vital-materialist creed as some-thing new in the world. But the fundamental insights are not new for everyone. They are ideas that . . . [undergird] an indigenous metaphysic: that matter is lively. We Dakota might say 'alive.' There is 'common materiality of all that is': we Dakota might say, 'We are all related. . . . Understanding these things can help transform how we humans see our place in the world, and therefore how we act" (199). As Western thinkers move to dismantle old analytic hierarchies privileging human beings, TallBear argues that indigenous frameworks are at a unique advantage because they never had those hierarchies to begin with. Indeed, Amerindian cos-mologies fueled the so-called ontological turn in anthropology associated with South Americanists like Viveiros de Castro (2014) and Descola (2013), who use Amerindian cosmologies as points of departure toward furthering an ambitious anthropological framework. Viveiros de Castro (2014) explicitly frames his proj-ect as a decolonial enterprise.

TallBear builds on the work of Vine Deloria Jr. (2001) to write about an "indig-enous metaphysic: that is, an understanding of the intimate knowing relatedness of all things" (2016,191). The indigenous metaphysic proposed by TallBear would thus not only recognize the inherent importance of materials, but also their abil-ity to recognize a "soul" or "spirit." In Western thought, the idea of "souls" or "spir-its" crosses an uncomfortable boundary between science and religion, but this boundary has little relevance in indigenous thought. Efrain's story illustrates this point.

It was, it was . . . everything was all mixed up there and . . . in the night, I tell my wife, when I woke up, I tell her, "hey, . . . help me pray." And when she heard that I was speaking in tongues like that and I was praying, she said, you are not my husband, she said. "Why not?" I asked. "Because you are not my husband. You are the evil spirit who is inside you," she said. "Why do you say that?" I said, and we went outside, to the kitchen. "You are the evil spirit," she said. "How can it be?" I said. "Yes, you are the evil spirit." "How can you prove it?" "This is how I prove it." And she hit me, my wife, she hit me here, but, really, really hard. And I said to her, "hit me so that the evil spirit that you say is inside me will leave." Then she said, "Son, come here," she said to my 12-year-old son. "Son, come see your dad, come see your dad. He is not your dad," she said, "Where is he?" She says, "Look, see how he's grabbed my hair," and she says, "Hit him." And so my son hits me and that's how I got this black eye.

Efrain ran into the woods after his son hit him, and he spent the night there. When he came home the next day, he found his house empty, save for his pet cardinal birds. The mated pair had a chick, and Efrain began conversing with them. He took the birds to his parents' home.

So I arrived at my mom's. I arrived at my mom's and I say, "Mommy . . ."
[and she says] "Why is your face like that? Who hit you?" she says.
And I said "Well, my wife and my son."
"How can that be?"
"Yes."
"Why, then?"
And my little sister, [she says] "Oh, brother, what is happening to you is not normal," she says. "Why? Why are you talking to the birds?"
She could hear me talking to them, and I said, "the baby, the baby folds his wings, both of them . . . he folds them like this . . . so they want to fly." And he turned like this . . . he turned back and started to say that they are going to fly, to fly. You fly, he said, and do not tell them it is me, said the baby.
And I, what could I do? I started to talk with my dad, but he couldn't understand me. And with my sister, but she couldn't understand me. And . . . well . . .
My little sister says, "brother, I am very sorry," she says, "but I am going to set your cardinals free."
"Why?"
"I'm going to set them free, brother. Poor birds, would you like to be locked up the way they are locked up?" She says.
"No," I say.
"So let them go, let them go and let them live like we live," she says.
With tears, with tears and pain, I let them go. But so you see, they didn't go far. They stayed near the house and started to sing and sing, all three of them. Yes. Then

my wife left, and they started to find a van so they could bring me here. . . . [the birds] come from God, because I fed them, but I had them locked in a cage, and it is not right to keep them locked up. Just like I'm locked up, right? I am fed, but I do not have freedom.

The idea that objects not only have agency, but also spirit, allows one to see the power of the uniform in a new light. Considering what we already know about Efrain's worldview, we know that the uniform, like the birds, is similar to other invisible beings inhabiting Efrain's world. Rather, invisible beings may not be invisible after all. It may simply be that they are visible to some actors and not to others.

An immediate argument against using TallBear's indigenous metaphysics to analyze the experiences of psychiatric patients in the psychiatric hospital is that the very idea of an indigenous metaphysic runs the risk of reifying essentialist constructions of "the indigenous." Surely, one would argue, the experiences of North American Indians—the perspective from which DeLoria and TallBear make their argument—are distinct from those of Yucatec Maya people. Second, it is not safe to assume that every patient in the ward is Yucatec Maya. To the first challenge, the easiest recourse is to locate an indigenous metaphysic in Maya tradition itself, if there is one.

Is there a distinct Maya metaphysic? The Maya concept of *iknal* (Hanks 1990; Castillo Cocom, Rodriguez, and Ashenbrender 2017), introduced in chapter 2, comes to mind. Iknal refers to an extension of the self into a spatial presence that can include objects. One's iknal can linger in place in one's absence, and Maya conceptions of health are closely tied to the maintenance of balance among the body, its spirits, and its multiple spatial extensions. Javier Hirose explains it in this way: "The spaces occupied by the human being in the cosmos—the home, the *solar*, the *milpa*, the town, and the world—constitute extensions of the body, while the spatial-temporal location of the human being in relationship with these spaces determines the condition of illness or health" (2008, 1). Moreover, Castillo Cocom and colleagues' (2016) work on iknal in the context of ethnoexodus implies that this bodily extension inhabits objects themselves. One's iknal may be present in a favorite chair, an often-used hammock, a beloved toy. For them, iknal is a bond in the form of spatial presence.

This perspective certainly seems to echo the idea of "an understanding of the intimate knowing relatedness of all things" espoused in TallBear's and Deloria's indigenous metaphysic, which can be understood as an indigenous ontology. In contrast to the decidedly secular ontology of new materialisms in the work of scholars such as Jane Bennett, indigenous ontologies recognize what TallBear calls "spirit." TallBear's work presents a useful framework for thinking through Yucatan's indigenous ontologies without subjugating them to Euro-American interpretations that trace their genealogies back to Deleuzian immanence (Viveiros de

Castro) or Foucauldian subjectivity (Rose), though an analysis informed by either of these would be valuable as well.

Even if one accepts that Yucatec Maya ontologies are similar enough to the indigenous metaphysic proposed by TallBear and Deloria for a productive reading of these data using their framework, not every patient in the ward is Maya or even from Yucatan. Why would an indigenous ontological perspective be useful for understanding the experiences of people who are not indigenous? A first counterargument to this suggestion would be to note that this is already being done and to point to the emergence of the kind of programmatic ontological anthropology visible in the work of Eduardo Viveiros de Castro (2014). Viveiros de Castro uses Amazonian Amerindian cosmologies to describe indigenous philosophies as part of a self-described mission to decolonize anthropological thought. A related counterargument can be seen in recent critiques by both Kim TallBear (2010) and Zoe Todd (2016) of the invisibility of indigenous thought in other ontological currents in the field of science, technology, and society (STS). TallBear writes of the new materialisms: "Indigenous thinkers have important contributions to make. . . . We should remember that not everyone needs to summon a new analytical framework or needs to renew a commitment to the 'the vitality of [so-called] things.' Indigenous standpoints that never constructed hierarchies in quite the same way can and should be at the forefront of this new ethnographic and theoretical work" (2016, 193). Likewise, of Latour's actor-network theory, indigenous feminist anthropologist Zoe Todd (Métis/otipemisiw) notes that despite commonalities between indigenous worldviews that perceive the agency and sentience of nonhuman actors as key innovations of the ontological turn, indigenous scholars who have been using similar frameworks for decades have been routinely ignored. In chapter 2, I argue that identity categories are fluid in contemporary Yucatan, and, ultimately, Las Lomas should be understood as a manifestation of the colonial matrix of power. In harmony with the decolonial acknowledgment of epistemic plurality, an indigenous metaphysics presents a useful way of thinking through the ontology of the psychiatric ward.

Iknal's temporality, characterized by presence in absence (my iknal remains in my empty chair long after I'm gone), is very similar to the concept of the Zona del Estar. Like iknal, Zona del Estar is characterized by a temporality of the present. Also, like iknal, Zona del Estar bridges two different states of being—in the case of the former, it allows for the existence of persons in material objects. In the latter case, it bridges the space between zones of being and nonbeing in the colonial matrix of power. However, iknal is a sociotemporal connection to spaces and objects. It offers a metaphysics where Zona del Estar offers a temporality. The patients inside the acute ward of Las Lomas can be understood to inhabit the Zona del Estar as a state of time, as they exist between the madness of nonbeing and the sanity of being. Iknal, as a more dynamic metaphysical force, can better elucidate what it means to exist in this zone.

The choice to read through stories like those of Claudina, or Efrain, or Candy, using indigenous scholarship and indigenous ontologies, is certainly a deliberate political choice; however, this scholarship also presents an analytical framework that is well suited to the ontological patterns expressed in their stories. I build on this to argue that in this particular setting, relationality is key to understanding the experiences of patients who find themselves committed at Las Lomas.

BROKEN BONDS

Efrain was the first intensive care patient I had ever interviewed at Las Lomas. Personal chemistry can make interviews particularly successful or particularly unsuccessful. Efrain and I clicked; our conversation was fluid and friendly, and at the end of the interview he wished me well with what appeared to be genuine warmth. Still somewhat giddy from this surprisingly pleasant experience in an increasingly depressing summer, I went back to Dr. Tun's office, where she was sitting at her desk, her laptop out. Efrain was not her patient, because Seguro Popular patients are segregated by gender, but Efrain, with his purple eye and talk of demon possession, had interested the psychiatrists on the ward. When I entered her office, she looked up from her work.

"How was it?"

I smiled. "It was good, I think."

She smiled back and cocked her head slightly. "He's still psychotic, right?"

"Well, he still thinks his birds were speaking to him," I replied.

She nodded knowingly and said nothing, returning to her work on the screen. Was he still psychotic? I did not think so. As a Maya man and as a Pentecostal Christian, his worldview already included the existence of the devil and the reality of demonic possession. It granted birds the ability to speak. The possibility of magic was real. It seemed to me that whether Efrain still believed he had been possessed, or whether he believed birds could converse with humans, was not really all that relevant to whether he saw himself as healthy or sick. Rather, his story presents an opportunity to appreciate the usefulness and importance of relationality in this analysis.

What is meant by relationality? Butler's call for a bodily ontology may bear some examination here. Relationality is not merely about how one thing is related to another, but rather about the ways in which people like those at Las Lomas experience ruptures in their relationships to humans and nonhumans alike. Claudina can adore her wounds as something external to herself because at the heart of her betrayal of her own body (through self-harm and her suicide attempt), there is a relational rupture in what she perceives to be her body and spirit. For Efrain, this rupture begins in his differences with his wife and ends with his experience of demonic possession. His experience is marked by multiple ruptures: with his family, with his beloved birds, with his clothing. Rupture is also at the heart of

Candy's story in the way her very self ruptures and gives way to her alter-ego, Anthony. These ruptured relationships characterize each patient's experience of illness. And what is a ruptured relationship if it is not a rupture in balance like that described earlier by Hirose? If iknal itself is described as a bond—another relationship—in the form of spatial presence, the multiple broken, mended, twisted, and renewed bonds described in these patients' stories point to a suffering iknal.

The relational dimensions of illness became evident in each of my interviews with patients in the acute ward. When I asked each of the twenty-five patients to describe what a sick person was, time and again patients would speak about illness in terms of the sick person's ability to function as a social being. The excerpts below are from interviews in which the question, *What is a sick person like?* was posed to each respondent.

BEATRIZ: What is a sick person?
CANDY: Well, someone who doesn't care what they do, who doesn't realize they are sick, who doesn't understand she is being told to obey for her own good.
BEATRIZ: So, this thing that happens to you with Anthony and Lupita, is this a sickness?
CANDY: It is.
BEATRIZ: What else characterizes a sick person?
CANDY: Sometimes they don't do what they are told. They are stubborn. Rude. They throw tantrums.

BEATRIZ: What is a sick person?
EFRAIN: A sick person doesn't think things through. They say things, or cry for any little thing, or, maybe they can't walk, they're sick. You feel sad all the time, is a sick person, they feel like, like an ogre, is a sick person.

Candy and Efrain, whose experiences are explored in this chapter, both describe illness and health in terms of how people act toward others. They were not unique in this. Illness was frequently described in relational terms. Some patients differentiated illness from mental illness:

ROSA: A sick person is someone who screams, who falls apart, whose nervios are easily altered. Someone with a cold is also a sick person. . . . The ones who are mentally ill are the ones who scream, who curse, scream, hit. The ones who are just sick don't do those things.
LUCIA: A sick person is a person who drinks alcohol or gets high. Who kills people, or hurts people. Who is violent.

In each of these answers, patients distinguish between physical illness and mental illness in different ways. Several patients invoked nervios, the quintessential culture-bound syndrome. A condition that is present throughout Latin America and the Caribbean, nervios is characterized by a combination of physical and emotional symptoms, particularly loss of emotional control. It has been described as a condition in which patients experience irritability, shakiness, dizziness, loss of consciousness, moodiness, crying, anger, and rage (Guarnaccia, DeLaCancela, and Carrillo 1989; Guarnaccia et al. 1996). However, in all these instances, the symptoms described are problematic because they cause behavior that is considered antagonizing by others.

Nerio, however, draws an interesting distinction between illness, mental illness, nervios, and substance abuse.

NERIO: The person who is just sick has nervios. Nervios is something that is in the blood. Everyone has it, but when people drink too much their nerves get weak and they want to kill themselves. I'm sick, but I'm not crazy, I just suffer from nervios.

For Nerio, nervios is not a mental illness, even though its symptoms may be emotional. Hence, *he is sick, but he is not crazy*. "Crazy" is incurable. Sickness is not. At first glance, one might argue that this description of illness is not relational. However, suicide and suicide attempts are relational, even if the relation being antagonized is a relation to one's own self.

OUTSIDE IN

May has always been the hottest month of the year. It is the end of the dry season, and the air tastes like dust. When I go to wipe sweat from my forehead, my hand comes back smudged with dirt. The rains will come soon enough, but in the meantime, we live with the heat. In 2012, the fans were broken in the acute ward; the patients lay sweating on black rubber mattresses, staring out the open windows onto the trees of the ward's inner courtyard. The heart of madness is in the acute ward, the place where patients in psychosis languish alongside the ones who attempted suicide and those suffering from eating disorders. I arrived at Las Lomas in early May that year, as soon as the spring semester at my university ended.

I introduced Eva in chapter 1; she was one of the first patients I encountered during my time inside Las Lomas's acute care ward. As I explained, she was a recently graduated biologist with a skeptical, scientific mind, who had been working in a university laboratory when a family conflict had triggered a temporary, stress-induced psychotic break. She was brought to the hospital wearing an evening gown and full makeup in the middle of the day, and she was speaking incoherently about a curse on her hand and the astrological connections between current and historical events. Dr. Tun was fascinated with her case.

DR. TUN: Eva, about this curse, you say it made your arm hurt, when did that start?

EVA: It's just an expression, you know, calling it a curse. I think it's more of a psychological question. All that pressure that I couldn't get out any other way, I got it out that way. We're not talking about magic here, it's just a way of saying things.

DR. TUN: Okay, so what is the relationship between the curse, the computer, and your sister?

EVA: Well, my mom and my sister told me that my hand was going to rot from using the computer so much.

Dr. Tun was always fascinated by the specific content of patient delusions. For her, there was significance to the fact that some of Eva's symptoms had somatized into pain in her arm. She was fascinated by Eva's dual discourse, which contained both magical elements—the curse—but logically dismissed them when she said, "We're not talking about magic here."

It is also possible that Eva understood very well that talking of curses and astrology would prolong her confinement. During the interview just quoted, Eva went on to explain what drove her to push herself to finish her degree and develop a professional career.

EVA: My family wants me to get well because they want me to help support them financially.

DR. TUN: How did this come about, Eva? Why do they expect this from you?

EVA: My father told me, right before he died. He said I had to complete my studies and help my family. My father saw a gift in me, he always saw both sides of the coin. My mother only ever saw the bad side, but my father was a very wise man who always saw the best in me.

DR. TUN: But, Eva, have you ever wanted anything else for yourself?

EVA: No, never. My father was very wise. He have me a mission, and I have to complete it. I am so tired, but I made a commitment. I love my family. My father, and my family.

Both Dr. Tun and her resident, Carolina, remarked on how quickly Eva's psychosis had subsided. "Her thinking has structured itself very quickly," Carolina remarked, "the psychosis remitted in two days." However, when her mother came in to speak with Dr. Tun after visiting hours, she had a different perspective. When Dr. Tun asked her whether she thought Eva was back to her old self, Eva's mother bit her lip for a moment and slowly shook her head.

"She still has a ways to go," she said.

"Why do you say that?" Dr. Tun asked.

She hesitated again. "Look," she started. "I don't know if I should tell you this. But just before we brought her here she got in the water back home. You know we live in Chelem. She went in the ocean, and she saw her father. And just now, during visiting hours, she was talking about it."

Dr. Tun adjusted her eyeglasses, thoughtful. "Do you believe she is hiding symptoms so that we release her?"

Eva's mother shook her head with a grieved expression. "I don't know. But she is very bright, it's possible."

After Eva's mother left, Dr. Tun turned to me and Carolina. "This story gets more and more interesting," she said, as I tried to jot down her words. "Eva deposits in her body all her reasons to get away from her family. She is living through a struggle between her personal needs and desires and her responsibilities towards her family. This young woman is fragile because she lives a constant fragmentation. The mission she is so passionately pursuing keeps her grounded in reality, and without it she falls into psychosis. I wonder if she has not been psychotic for quite a long time."

Eva was transferred out of the acute care ward before I was able to interview her. Whether her psychotic break had been the result of a fragile balance broken by her feuding family, or from the stress of balancing a demanding job in the sciences with her family responsibilities, or something else entirely, will remain unknown. However, Eva's discourse, recorded through observation of her conversations with her medical provider, reveals a driven young woman whose discourse expresses both magical thinking and scientific skepticism. She knows enough to say, firmly, that the "curse" she feels in her arm is not magical—an expression, in different words, of Dr. Tun's interpretation that the pain in her arm is connected to the pressure of supporting her family and building her career. Within two days of being committed, Eva was able to express that the frightening connections she had been making between historical and astronomical events were the result of her psychosis. Yet, according to her mother, she continued to believe her father had appeared to her in the waves of the sea.

In this book, I have so far described the ways in which Las Lomas and the people it purports to help are interwoven in the colonial matrix of power. I have described the emergence of the Zona del Estar as a temporality bridging the gap between madness and reason, being and nonbeing. In chapter 6, I have explored the most irreducible unit of the psychiatric encounter: the intersubjective experiences of the patients Las Lomas is trying to treat. Specifically, I have engaged with the lived experiences of several patients I encountered in my time at Las Lomas who were struggling with crippling symptoms. All were hospitalized inside the acute care ward, and most would be considered psychotic by their psychiatrists, though by the time they agreed to speak to me they had been judged capable to give informed consent.

Throughout this book, I have made the argument that Las Lomas is a manifestation of the colonial matrix of power. But what that means for the people locked in its wards, especially those in its most cruel space, the acute care ward, has not been thoroughly explored. I have delved into the stories of individuals who were patients inside the acute care ward at Las Lomas, and I have considered the ways in which the ward functions as an institution of coloniality. In some ways, one can identify parallels between Eva and Manuela, whose interaction with Dr. Pacheco I analyze in chapter 5, as they negotiated an acceptable truth. While in chapter 5 I argued that "the truth" was less relevant than "the believable" as a measure of improvement in the psychiatric institution, in this chapter I access the truths and realities as they are experienced by patients in the acute care ward. If psychiatric institutions exist as way of disciplining unruly minds and bodies, delving into the heart of madness is important for understanding the world at the edge of experience (Jenkins 2015).

Silvia, a woman in her early twenties, was also committed to Las Lomas in the oppressive heat of May. We learned that she had been committed over the weekend when we came in to work on Monday morning. When I met her on May 28, she came in for morning consultation, asking to be released before she had even sat down in front of Dr. Tun's desk. Silvia was from Tizimin, a small, cattle-ranching city in Yucatan's easternmost region about four hours' drive from Merida. "I have to return to Tizimin," she said, urgency in her voice, "please, I have to return my students' workbooks."

Over the next few days, I had the opportunity to observe the evolution and transformation of Silvia's symptoms as Dr. Tun continued to treat and monitor her progress. Once Silvia agreed to sit for her morning consultation with Dr. Tun, it quickly became apparent that she was in the grips of a powerful and terrifying delusion.

DR. TUN: Silvia, why are you here?

SILVIA: I don't know. I think they put something in my *frijol con puerco* [rice and beans]. They have been trying to poison me.

DR. TUN: Who is "they," Silvia? Your family?

SILVIA: Yes, and the nurses, too. They keep calling me "rabbit." Can I leave? Can you release me so I can go home?

DR. TUN: I thought they were trying to poison you at home.

SILVIA: No, no. I feel better now. I really do.

DR. TUN: This morning, when I came to your bed, you said something about your sister. What did you say you were concerned about?

SILVIA: Oh, that. Yes. I'm concerned, I'm very concerned. My sister wants to steal my heart.

DR. TUN: Really? And how is she planning on doing that?

SILVIA: With a surgery. She's going to extract it with surgery.

DR. TUN: Surgery? Is she a doctor? A surgeon?

SILVIA: No, but you are. That's why I'm here. That's why I was brought here. You're going to take my heart. And my eyes, too.

DR. TUN: But, Silvia, why would we do that? Why would we want to take your heart and eyes?

SILVIA: To give them to my sister! And then you're going to give me *her* heart and eyes. It's what she wants, but it won't help her. She wants my heart but if she takes it, it won't be any good. It won't do what she wants it to do.

DR. TUN: What does she want with your heart?

SILVIA: My heart is pure and good, that's why she wants it. So she can get into heaven.

The story that followed was consistent, if perhaps outlandish. Silvia said she owed her sister money, and her sister had demanded her heart and eyes as payment. She believed she had been possibly drugged and brought to Las Lomas, where this surgery to switch her heart and eyes with those of her sister was supposed to take place. One day, she came into the consultation room with a solution: Doña Isabel, another patient on the ward, had offered her a job.

SILVIA: But listen, you should let me go! Doña Isabel is going to help me! I have a job offer! I can pay my sister back!

DR. TUN: Doña Isabel offered you a job?

SILVIA: Yes! I'm going to take care of a baby. She asked me if I wanted to go with her, and I said yes.

DR. TUN: But Silvia, Doña Isabel isn't leaving yet. She's going to be here a while. Tell me more about your sister's plan. When did she come up with it? Why do you think she has this plan?

SILVIA: She told me! She told me, on March 26. She threatened me. I have this blanket; it has *The Little Mermaid* on it. My sister wants me to look like the little mermaid.

DR. TUN: So you want to look like the little mermaid?

SILVIA: No! That's not healthy. *She*, my sister, she wants me to waste away to look like that. Listen, did you do it already? Did you give me her heart?

DR. TUN: No, we didn't. Silvia, we will not do surgery on you here.

SILVIA: So can I leave? Can I go home?

DR. TUN: Not today. We ran some tests, we would like to see the results.

SILVIA: Okay, okay. But listen. I want you to help me. I don't want you to take my heart. If I were a doctor, I would be saving lives, not harming them. I would do my job, and help people.

DR. TUN: Silvia, I can assure you, we will not do anything to harm you. We will help you.

SILVIA: So I can leave, then?

DR. TUN: No, not today. We will talk again tomorrow.

Carolina took Silvia back to the ward, and Dr. Tun reflected on the case. "Her thinking is fragmented, but the delusion is consistent," she said, "and now Doña Isabel is offering her a job. But you know, all of these things she's saying. They're strange. All of that, her family hears her and they hear *locura*. The sister concludes, *my sister is mad, saying I'm going to take her eyes.*" When encountering patients using the kind of discourse Silvia used, biomedically oriented psychiatrists like Dr. Castro or even Dr. Pacheco generally noted that the patient was suffering from delusion, but rarely took the time to analyze the content of the so-called delusions. Dr. Tun, however, as a psychoanalytically oriented psychiatrist, always found these delusions ripe for analysis, and she paid careful attention to their content as she made her diagnoses.

Silvia's delusion was unremitting over the next several days. Dr. Tun and Carolina puzzled over her case. The exchange that follows took place a few days later. Silvia once again expressed concerns about her sister wanting to steal her heart, but when Dr. Tun queried her further by asking her how she thought this might happen, this time Silvia thought for a moment, and replied, "Well, no, that's impossible. She can't take my heart."

DR. TUN: Hmm, I don't know. I don't think it's schizoaffective because she doesn't meet all the criteria. Yes, her ideas indicate delirium, but she's not having auditory hallucinations.

CAROLINA: She shakes her head a lot, as if she were hearing voices. She has something she wants to say, but something is stopping her. She thinks she is being persecuted.

DR. TUN: Yes, she's psychotic. But I'm not convinced it's schizoaffective. She doesn't meet the criteria for schizoaffective or for schizophrenia, not completely.

Dr. Tun continued:

Auditory hallucinations predominate in schizophrenia, that's not the case here. That's where the affective dimension comes in. She's obsessed with the workbooks because she is afraid she is going to get in trouble. I think this was a task she was supposed to complete, but wasn't able to, so now she can't let it go. She's fixated. Her entire delirium is fixated on this fear of punishment—that someone is going to inject her, someone is going to take her heart—but she's capable of making a rational, logical argument, right? She's afraid her sister wants to take her heart, but she also just told us that logically, that's impossible. She also told us today she is happy, and she can't understand why. She feels an overwhelming desire to say hello to everyone, even people she doesn't know, but the desire perplexes her. She is trying hard to use logic to understand what is happening, so we can rule out schizophrenia. This behavior all leads me to think she has some kind of bipolar disorder. We don't yet know which one, perhaps a sub-classification.

Dr. Tun's primary objective in the context of these conversations is to explain as carefully and deliberately as possible her diagnostic process to her resident, Carolina. However, reflecting on both Silvia's conversation with Dr. Tun and Dr. Tun's own interpretation of Silvia's story, one can appreciate the mechanisms of madness that both gives the outsider a glimpse into Silvia's world and seeks to categorize her experience into a diagnostic category. Two distinct experiences are at play from two dramatically different viewpoints: Dr. Tun's experience assessing and diagnosing Silvia's symptoms, and Silvia's experience of confinement and persecution. In the first instance, Dr. Tun recognizes Silvia's madness when she says, after their initial meeting, "Her family hears her and they hear *locura*." Silvia's delusion, turned on her immediate family, results in her confinement. In the second, it is impossible to truly access Silvia's experience: she fears for her life, and her fear centers on a medical procedure. Her confinement in a hospital further confirms her fears, as hospitals are locations for surgeries.

We learned more about Silvia from her family. Having completed vocational training in child development, Silvia worked at a child-care center. She helped her mother with her small *panuchos* business.[7] Her sister had loaned her some money that she could not immediately repay, and this had led to arguments. However, no one seemed to know how she had become ill. She started obsessing, "saying nonsense," and becoming increasingly fearful that she was being poisoned. Her family took her to see a local doctor, and he had referred her to Las Lomas for treatment.

Time went on. Dr. Tun continued to puzzle over Silvia's diagnosis. Silvia continued to believe her sister was trying to take her heart and eyes and that she was being poisoned. This concern over poisoning led her to refuse meals, and her condition rapidly worsened. After several days of observation, Dr. Tun finally decided to prescribe ECT. Although I was familiar with the efficacy of ECT for treating medication-resistant depression, I had never heard of that particular treatment, which is considered a treatment of last resort in the United States, being used to treat psychosis.

When I asked Dr. Tun about her decision to send Silvia to ECT, she spoke with conviction: "ECT is more humane than force-feeding. This patient hasn't been eating, her condition is rapidly deteriorating. ECT will bring her out of her psychotic state and make her more compliant." At the time of my research, Las Lomas was the only facility in the region where this treatment could be accessed. On average, ECT was administered to three to six patients a week, often to patients like Silvia who were refusing food because of paranoid or psychotic symptoms. Although I could appreciate Dr. Tun's concern regarding Silvia's refusal to eat, I knew that Silvia had been eating the food her family had brought in for her, and I could not help but wonder whether it would have been better to allow Silvia to eat food she could trust and allow the antipsychotics to take effect. For Dr. Tun, compliance was a measurement of improvement. Allowing Silvia to eat her family's food would encourage Silvia's delusion that the hospital was trying to poison her, making this option unacceptable.

The morning following her first ECT treatment, Silvia's delirium began to change, though it did not immediately remit. The confusion that followed as a side effect of the treatment made diagnosis more challenging. Her previously cheerful mood evaporated into deep sadness. The presence of an IV line in her arm frightened her, and she expressed concern that hospital staff had infected her with the AIDS virus. She no longer seemed to remember a conflict with her sister, and her concern with her students' workbooks faded as well. Instead, when Dr. Tun asked her about her life, Silvia began telling us about her mother's panucho business, making an unbelievable claim that her family earned 10,000 pesos (about USD $5,300 in 2012, a substantial amount of money) per day. Dr. Tun exclaimed in disbelief:

DR. TUN: I don't believe it! I will hang up my doctor's coat and go make panuchos! How much do you make a week?
SILVIA: About 7,000 pesos.
DR. TUN: Well, hold on. That isn't logical. Let's add it up.

Silvia attempted to add up the amount of money her family made selling panuchos every week, but she was unable to keep track of the numbers. After a minute or so, Dr. Tun stopped her.

DR. TUN: So you all are wealthy, then!
SILVIA: Our panuchos are delicious, we have a secret recipe.
DR. TUN: A secret? Can you tell me what the secret is?
SILVIA: No, no! My mother will get angry. No, come and try them instead.
DR. TUN: I can't go all the way to Tizimin just to eat panuchos!
SILVIA: Where are we?
DR. TUN: We're in Merida.

At this point some of the effects of the ECT treatment had become clear—for instance, Silvia knew we were in Merida prior to her treatment, but had she lost her sense of place after the treatment. After this exchange, Dr. Tun and Carolina analyzed her progress. Dr. Tun reflected:

Well, she's certainly more organized. Since last week, we've been seeing her with disorganized thinking, her affect has been expansive. Now, her ideas are expansive. I mean, she's better, but the psychosis has not remitted. She has grandiose ideas, like that her family makes 10,000 pesos in a week selling panuchos—those must be the best panuchos in Yucatan—and she has a secret. So her ideas are still showing some delirium. Her affect has certainly changed. She was very cheerful before, now she seems sad and withdrawn. I really do suspect this may have been a first manic episode with delirium. Her problems with calculations and abstract thinking can be explained by the ECT, so we will give her the benefit of the doubt there and say they are likely temporary.

The next day, following her second ECT treatment, Silvia's condition changed dramatically. She did not seem so confused, her mood improved, and her thinking became, in psychiatric parlance, more organized. She no longer held on to the secret recipe.

DR. TUN: So, Silvia, I wanted you to share the secret ingredient with me! The one in your mother's panuchos!

SILVIA: You want to know the secret? Okay, I'll tell you. It starts with F. Guess.

DR. TUN: No, tell me.

SILVIA: It's flour! It changes the texture of the *masa*.

DR. TUN: So how much do you sell?

SILVIA: Well, it really depends on the day, but I'd say we usually sell about 8 kilos, sometimes 10 on Sundays.

DR. TUN: And how much money does your family make selling panuchos?

SILVIA: Well, again, it depends, but probably about 800 pesos.

Silvia now seemed to be firmly grounded in reality. When Dr. Tun asked her if anyone was trying to hurt her, she denied any concerns. Carolina then followed up with another question:

CAROLINA: Silvia, tell me. Do you think it is possible for someone to take your heart out? For someone to switch it?

SILVIA: Sure, it's possible. But you would die!

The fear that her heart would be surgically removed had finally remitted. The psychosis was gone. With that, the interview ended, as did Silvia's ECT treatment. She was transferred to the long-term ward, where after a few days of observation, she was able to return home.

I never had the opportunity to interview Silvia, so I will never know what she thought about her situation or her experiences of delusion. Her own experience is inaccessible to us. In many ways, the experiences of people who suffer from mental illness, or anyone for that matter, are always inaccessible. Silvia's discourse, recorded over two weeks of observing her conversations with Dr. Tun, interweaves worries about money, feelings of responsibility toward work, and familial conflict with a fear of bodily harm. Eva's and Silvia's stories illustrate the interaction of worlds inhabited by patients and doctors. Eva's mission, her father's presence, the material objects and body parts of Silvia's obsession, meet Dr. Tun's diagnostic interpretation and the ECT machine, which ultimately brings an abrupt ending to alternative realities and beliefs deemed unacceptable.

The ECT machine also unveils the machinery of the colonial matrix of power: invisible beings and spatial presences lose their vibrancy under the weight of ECT and become fragile, vanishing memories. Eva's encounter with her father is hidden as she explains away the pain in her hand as somatization, not bewitchment. This is not to say that Silvia, Eva, or any of the people described in this chapter were not suffering from the voices, visions, and intrusive realities that came between them and the reality perceived by those of us in the zone of sanity. Rather, the way these experiences of delusion are understood, treated, and erased reveals the colonization of the psyche, the demand for the patient to let go of the beings, objects, and realities that inhabit the ward alongside them: in other words, an ontological colonization.

ONTOLOGY AND ITS DISCONTENTS

As I suggested earlier, the ontological turn in anthropology is not without its critics. Lucas Bessire's (2014) ethnography, *Behold the Black Caiman*, is a sustained critique of Vivierios de Castro and Descola's ontology, though other critiques have been made (Carrithers et al. 2010; Graeber 2015; Bond and Bessire 2014). Bessire (2014) argues that the ontological turn essentializes Amerindian cosmology, assuming its immutability and universalism. He connects this drive to locate an Amerindian cosmology with an anthropological fetishization of tradition, a drive that results in an unfounded perspectivism that misses the ways in which indigenous people—specifically, the Ayoreo of the northern Paraguayan Chaco—challenge these very notions. More seriously, Bessire argues, the current focus on Amerindian cosmology as a locus for thinking through the existence of multiple worlds—"one epistemology, multiple ontologies" (Viveiros de Castro 2012)—misses the reality of marginalization experienced by the very indigenous people whose cosmology has been so celebrated—"instead of jaguars who are humans, I found Indians who were animalized" (Bessire 2014, 15). Viveiros de Castro is making a universalist argument, although many decolonial scholars would call for epistemic plurality (Grosfoguel 2011b).[8] Bessire's critique is limited to one of several perspectives that could be considered within the broader theoretical perspective of the ontological turn. Nevertheless, the point is well taken: as I have discussed in various points throughout this book, Juan Castillo Cocom, a Yucatec Maya anthropologist, makes a similar critique in his own work on Maya identity.

I have briefly considered the appropriateness of engaging indigenous ontologies to examine the experiences of patients in the ward who may not be Maya. In chapter 2, I engaged with the troubled notion of Maya identity, noting the ways in which Yucatan's Maya heritage is a contested site at which notions of authenticity, cultural capital, and symbolic violence come together to produce an essentialized "Maya." This process of coming together, termed "ethnographic entrapment" (Simpson 2014; de Silva 2007), creates an entire class of people who do not fit into idealized stereotypes of people racialized as Maya (in terms of language, dress, religion, worldview) yet face the same systematic discrimination and social exclusion. Castillo Cocom argues that this phenomenon is directly related to the way the Mexican and Yucatecan states have used indigenous heritage and indigenous institutions strategically for the purposes of both bolstering economic development and—perhaps more importantly—controlling the region's indigenous people (Castillo Cocom 2005; Castillo Cocom and Ríos Luviano 2012). Bessire's portrayal of tradition as an ethnographic fetish is well supported in the work of Castillo Cocom, who places the responsibility for what he terms the "fifth creation of the Maya" squarely on the shoulders of anthropologists, linguists, historians, and archaeologists (2005, 133).

I, too, have grappled with the slippery notion of Maya identity (Reyes-Foster 2012, chapters 1 and 2 of this book), particularly as it affects people who do not conform to the fetishized version of the "traditional" Maya. In the hospital, this may include people like Efrain, who is Protestant and has a very low opinion of anything remotely "traditional," especially traditional cosmologies and medical practices. It might also include Claudina, who—as she herself states—does not eat "only tortillas and chile" like her grandmother, a "great wise woman"; and even Dr. Tun, who, despite having a Maya last name and all the physical attributes typically associated with Maya-ness, would never consider herself Maya. It is a troubling notion that the very framework used with decolonial intentions could represent yet another form of oppression and the possible symbolic erasure of people who are not indigenous enough to be Maya, but are too indigenous to have access to the kind of privileges enjoyed by white Yucatecans (Castillo Cocom 2005; Castillo Cocom and Ríos Luviano 2012; Rivera Cusicanqui 2010). Nevertheless, the passages presented earlier show the usefulness of this framework in thinking through the stories described in this chapter. Like my relationship with the white coat, the patients who generously shared their experiences, joys, and sorrows with me are also bound inextricably in complex and often painful ways to the visible and invisible, human and nonhuman beings that surround them.

7 · EPILOGUE

Quite frankly, if you aren't publishing your research shortly after you do it, you aren't writing anthropology anymore. You're recording history.
—Paul Rabinow, ANT 240, first-year anthropology seminar, UC Berkeley, fall 2004

What is happening at Las Lomas is what is happening in Mexico, *así, en chiquito*.
—Las Lomas psychiatrist, Merida, January 2017

Since the conclusion of my field research in Yucatan in 2013, I have frequently had the opportunity to present findings from my research in various academic settings. It was not rare that at the end of my talks, a hand would go up and someone in the audience, horrified by my descriptions of conditions on the ground, would ask, "Well, isn't there something to be done? Have you presented your findings to someone who can effect some kind of change in this institution?"

My response was usually measured. "I haven't needed to. The facility was subject to a human rights investigation shortly after I left it, and conditions on the ground have changed significantly."

In the years that have transpired since the last time I spent extensive periods of time inside its wards, Las Lomas saw three changes in leadership, an investigation by the Yucatan State Commission for Human Rights, the takeover of the facility by the federal government, and an influx of accompanying funding. The federal takeover of the institution was accompanied by predictable worker mobilization and grumblings from most of its staff. However, some positive changes have taken place. When I visited the institution in July 2016, I found that the wards had been remodeled and reorganized. Air conditioning had been installed, and each ward featured new, 55″ flat-screen televisions. The intensive care ward I had spent so many hours in had effectively been dismantled. New intensive care dormitories were added to the existing men's and women's wards, now known as *estancias* (lounges), instead of the medicalized *pabellones* (wards). New signage in Spanish and Yucatec Mayan had been added throughout the institution. The isolation room, where patients like Andrea, Lina, and Manuela had been interned, had been closed, and the space was now used for storage. With the exception of the two intensive care dormitories, which remained locked wards, the decorative masonry that had effectively turned the dormitories into cells had been knocked down; now the dormitories are separated from the ward reception areas only by a half wall. The wards were clean, cool, and comfortable. The dormitory bathrooms, even if still in the open, were functioning properly. The overpowering stench was gone. The beds in the dorms were made—no longer exposed rubber mattresses—and patients could come in and out of the wards as they wished. The ward building doors, formerly imposing black metal, had been replaced with frosted sliding glass. The art therapy room still featured beautiful artwork created by patients, but it was now also air-conditioned and freshly painted.

Some cracks in the veneer were visible. As Dr. Tun walked me through the occupational therapy building, I saw hospital staff enjoying the air-conditioning, watching television, reading magazines, and passing time. We walked up to another closed door and heard the unmistakable sounds of a telenovela through the door. Large spaces, such as the art therapy and occupational therapy buildings, are expensive to cool. When they are not in use, they are supposed to be closed, and the air conditioning is supposed to be turned off, yet we saw staff using these spaces for personal use.

For some, however, the most difficult administrative change was the closure of Las Lomas's ECT services. In response to what had been perceived as an overuse of ECT, the treatment was banned altogether. For many critics, this was tantamount to throwing the baby out with the bathwater—although some thought ECT was overused, it was seen as life-saving, life-changing treatment by others. Moreover, it was the only facility of its type in the peninsula. This meant that even people who may have benefited from ECT on an outpatient basis no longer had this service available to them.

The banning of ECT was a particular sticking point to the administration, which went out of its way to advertise this change. Headlines such as "No mas electrochoques a pacientes de Las Lomas" (No more electroshocks for patients at Las Lomas) appeared in local newspapers.[1] In one news report, the federal government representative overseeing Las Lomas's transition proudly proclaimed: "We are finished with scientific research in the hospital, and there will be no more electroshocks to our patients," indicating the beginning of a new era at the hospital. Alongside the banning of ECT, all scientific research taking place at Las Lomas was immediately suspended.

This new era was characterized by the implementation of the acclaimed "Hidalgo Model," a treatment model that aims to rehabilitate patients and enable them to reintegrate into society outside of the institution. This model certainly presents a move in the right direction for Mexican public psychiatry, as it stands in sharp contrast with the current model, which is, as has been described in this book, driven primarily by institutionalization. Under the Hidalgo Model, patients occupy "villas," independent shared houses where they live together with on-site medical supervision. They are provided with training and preparation to reintegrate into society (DRI 2011). In the state of Hidalgo, the first place where this model was implemented, halfway houses were constructed, allowing patients to move from the villas into the community. This initiative led to the closure of the state's only psychiatric hospital (Secretaría de Salud, 2007).

While living in villas in the Hidalgo Model, some patients are able to hold jobs outside the facility, and others earn money by doing odd jobs inside the facility. Disability Rights International observers were particularly impressed by one program that allowed patients to fully operate a hair salon inside the institution (2011, 29). However, there are currently few provisions for patients to actually integrate and live inside the broader community in other locations that have implemented versions of the Hidalgo Model, a challenge to the model noted by DRI observers (2011) who had inspected (and were frequently denied access to) the very few facilities operating under that model. Nevertheless, the Hidalgo Model seems to contain much promise, and it appears to be a far preferable approach to the current model of care.

However, the Hidalgo Model is not without criticism. It is explicitly intended for chronically ill, long-term patients. It is not intended for the treatment of acutely ill people during short-term stays, which represented the majority of hospital admissions at Las Lomas. The treatment model itself is new and not yet supported by scientific evidence. It is also not an adequate program for people who are mentally ill and under the custody of the criminal justice system. For example, in Cancun during the summer of 2017, a Russian neo-Nazi who suffered from schizophrenia was attacked by an angry mob and nearly lynched. The man killed one of his attackers during the incident and was subsequently arrested for murder. However, the severity of his illness necessitated hospitalization, and it was quickly discovered that the only facility in the entire region that would have been able to take him, Las Lomas, was no longer equipped to house a person diagnosed as criminally insane. The treatment philosophy at the institution had changed. The Hidalgo Model had come to Las Lomas to free its residents, but this meant no walls, no locks, and no criminals.

It is difficult to know what the future holds for Las Lomas. Some of the changes that have been made in the facility, particularly the infrastructural improvements, are unquestionably positive and have improved the quality of life of patients. The outcome of others, such as the suspension of ECT treatment and research activities, is unknown. Whether this particular iteration of the Hidalgo Model is an appropriate model for Las Lomas and Yucatan in general remains to be seen. Predictably, the transition to federal control has been accompanied by numerous obstacles and feuding, with both sides (state officials, former health secretaries and hospital directors, the local press, and the federal agency taking over the institution) accusing one another of corruption and embezzlement. Ironically, it seemed that the shift toward the Hidalgo model had finally succeeded in bringing doctors, nurses, and social workers to set their differences aside and work together to oppose the reorganization. One hundred hospital employees paralyzed the institution in October 2016 with a strike protesting changes in working conditions and the newly imposed hospital administration.

Nevertheless, as the takeover entered its second year, in March 2016, plans for the construction of a new inpatient facility made up entirely of Hidalgo Model–style villas were announced. If all goes according to plan, Las Lomas as an inpatient psychiatric facility will cease to exist. In summer 2017, some of the staunchest opponents of the new facility claimed that the money earmarked for its construction had already been embezzled. Construction on the new project, named Villas de Transición Hospitaliaria (Transitional Hospital Villas) and lauded by official state press releases as a "modern complex for mental health care," finally began on March 15, 2018.

The events at Las Lomas since the conclusion of my field research could support an entirely new manuscript—unfortunately, the hospital ban on research (and the fact that other Hidalgo Model institutions have restricted access to international observers such as DRI) makes this a difficult endeavor. The federal takeover of Las Lomas and its imminent closing beg the question: What is the relevance of the Las Lomas I studied to our understanding of Mexican psychiatry and the Mexican mental health system after such dramatic changes have taken place? What does it mean to write about confinement when the same institution that once confined patients to locked wards is now dedicated to tearing these wards down?

A colleague, one of several Las Lomas psychiatrists I had the opportunity to work with, met me for coffee in Merida in January 2017. After exchanging pleasantries and New Year's greetings, we talked about what was happening at Las Lomas. Reflecting on the turbulence of the times, my friend's head shook in wonder and dismay. "What is happening at Las Lomas is what is happening in Mexico, así, en chiquito [like this, in miniature]." This is because nothing in Mexico happens outside of politics—the federal entity that has taken over the institution, like all other federal entities, is directed by a person who is heavily connected in Mexican party politics. The takeover created new factions, new fights, new competing interests to replace the old. My friend was among those convinced that the takeover was characterized by widespread fraud and embezzlement. I cannot ascertain whether this is the case, but my friend's statement resonates: Mexico continues to go through transformations and unrest. Old factions and interests are being replaced by new ones. As Mexico has transformed under the neoliberalizing efforts of its leadership, Mexico today may appear unrecognizable to those who came of age in Mexico yesterday. What is happening at Las Lomas as the institution reaches the end of its life may be what is happening in Mexico, as the revolutionary state also reaches its own end.

In the nineteenth century, the old Hospital San Hipólito became the country's first modern mental asylum.[2] It was subsequently replaced in 1910 by Porfirio Diaz's modern dream, La Castañeda. In Yucatan, the old Franciscan hospital at La Mejorada provided care to the mad, first under Franciscan administration, then under the state government. This institution was closed to make way for the old Asilo Ayala in 1906, and this facility continued to operate, as previously described, until it was replaced by Las Lomas in 1978. Now, it appears that Las Lomas itself will be replaced by something newer and supposedly better, something more con-cordant with the Mexican state's contemporary vision of modernity.

Will the new villas present a new era for psychiatric patients in Yucatan? Will this new era change the dynamics of the coloniality of power that I have continu-ously returned to in this book? If history is any kind of teacher, if change and modernization always comes with its own colonial baggage—as accusations of corruption and embezzlement seem to suggest—then it is possible to argue that no, it is unlikely that things will change in substance, even if they change in form. Perhaps the future will prove me wrong—I certainly hope this is the case.

I began this epilogue with something Paul Rabinow, who taught the first gradu-ate anthropology course I ever took at Berkeley, said to our class during the fall 2004 term. The gap between research and publication is so wide that things change on the ground before they appear in print. It is one of the problems of the "ethnographic present," the ethnographic writing style that situates all writing in a permanent present tense, giving the impression that things never change, that culture remains static and stable. But by the same token, colonialism and its associ-ated power structures (patriarchy, heteronormativity, Judeo-Christianity, racism) have remained constant in Mexico for nearly 500 years. This portrait of an insti-tution in decline in a peripheral region of a troubled nation teases out the ways in which disparity is produced by more than social structure and individual agency. It exists in a universe at the center of which are the complex experiences of colonial subjects. Even if we can successfully argue that colonialism continues to define the current world order, what colonialism looks like has shifted and changed over time, and that change has not taken place without resistance. The colonial matrix of power is not a monolith but is, rather, a web, a collection of networks and relations created and recreated at multiple levels of social existence. This book, while describing a moment now passed, remains unfortunately timely.

In Merida, life goes on. Dr. Vasquez continues his suicide prevention efforts inside and outside the institution. Dr. Tun continues to balance her private prac-tice with teaching, research, and clinical work inside and outside of Las Lomas. Dr. Patrón was finally able to find a permanent position in a different public insti-tution and left Las Lomas. Dr. Castro and Dr. Pacheco continue to balance work at Las Lomas with their own private practices. Dr. Treviño, whom I last saw in July 2016, continues to see patients and teach medical students and residents; he recently celebrated sixty years of continuous service. The residents I worked with over my time at Las Lomas have graduated. One of them, the resident I refer to as Ana, was subsequently hired and remained at Las Lomas, while the others have returned to their home states.

I can say little about the patients who appear in this book. As I explained at the outset, several of the patients I describe here are composite characters. I can say they have all moved on and out of the institution. Some of them have returned and been released again. Several continue to visit the institution for outpatient treatment. Others remain involved in Dr. Vasquez's suicide prevention program. Of the people who were never psychiatric patients but whose stories found their way into this book, Chelito, the young woman whose son was stillborn in chapter 2, has gone on to have two healthy girls. She continues to reside in Yaxche' with her family. Doña Candelaria and her family are likewise doing well, and her children and nieces are now adults who have children of their own.

As for myself, though I continue to maintain close personal ties to Yucatan, in recent years my attention has shifted elsewhere. The research that led to the writing of *Psychiatric Encounters* took a toll on my emotional health. It was difficult to carry out and at times extraordinarily difficult to write. Witnessing the suffering of other human beings is draining work. At this juncture, it is hard to see how the publication of this book will impact Las Lomas for better or for worse. What I do within it, however, is to consider Las Lomas as part of a Mexico that has an enduring and inherent colonial society. The colonial matrix of power manifests itself in other ways, yet madness pushes boundaries, troubles assumptions, and challenges beliefs about human nature, rationality, and reality. I have sought to evoke a new understanding of the ways in which coloniality shapes the existence of some of society's most vulnerable people, and so produces disparity. As Mexico's neoliberal path continues to unfold, this understanding is more pressing than ever before.

ACKNOWLEDGMENTS

This book was a long time in the making, and it would not have been possible without the support of many people over nearly ten years of work. My first debt of gratitude is to Lenore Manderson, editor of the Medical Anthropology: Health, Inequality, and Social Justice series at Rutgers University Press. Her early enthusiasm for the project, precise feedback, and meticulous reading made this book what it is today. Likewise, Kim Guinta, executive editor at Rutgers University Press, remembered our early conversations when this book was beginning to take shape and easily convinced me this series would be the right home for *Psychiatric Encounters*. I am grateful to them both for their faith in this project, and in me. Two anonymous reviewers also provided invaluable feedback that greatly strengthened the manuscript.

The research on which this book was supported by a number of financial sources. Research conducted during the doctoral work period was variously supported by the U.S. Department of Education's summer Foreign Language and Area Studies fellowship, a UC Berkeley Center for Latin American Studies Tinker Grant, and a U.S. State Department Fulbright-Hays Doctoral Dissertation Research Abroad grant. Subsequent research in Yucatan was supported by University of Central Florida startup funds. The University of Central Florida Department of Anthropology generously supported various aspects of the book-writing and production process, most notably through financial support of indexing and image publication permissions. I am especially grateful to Tosha Dupras, my chair in the Department of Anthropology at the University of Central Florida, who has been a source of great support during the writing and publication process.

I am indebted to many colleagues, collaborators, and friends in Mexico. Gaspar Baquedano Lopez has played a major role as a collaborator, mentor, and friend for over ten years, providing invaluable advice and intellectual engagement. Without Gaspar, this research would simply not have been possible. Likewise, Mercy Tut Rivero's thoughtful commentary helped me interpret much of what I witnessed on the ground. I am extremely grateful for my family in Merida, most notably the help and support extended by Graciela Cortés Camarillo, Claudia Chapa Cortés, and David Reyes Aguiar. Seidy Tun Hoo, Jorge Tun Hoo, and the extended Tun Chan family have been dear friends for many years.

This manuscript benefited greatly from the careful reading and feedback of many friends and colleagues. Deanna Barenboim, Gabriela Raquel Ríos, Katie Hendy, Rebecca Galemba, Vannia Smith-Oka, Adrienne Pine, and Elizabeth Farfán-Santos read and provided valuable guidance on various chapters during the manuscript-drafting process. Jennifer Richardson Branting generously read the entire manuscript prior to submission to Rutgers University Press. I am also indebted to Xochiquetzal Marsilli-Vargas and the Emory University SPANPORT Lecture Series and Ludek Broz and the Society for Czech Anthropology's Ernst Gellner Seminar Series for inviting me to present my research in Atlanta and Prague as this book was coming into being. The conversations and feedback received at both venues were invaluable. I am especially grateful for a conversation with Karen Stolley at Emory and her suggestion of the idea of *Zona del Estar* during my visit to deliver a lecture for the SPANPORT Lecture Series. Kim Tall-Bear shared an unpublished version of her chapter, "Beyond the Life/Not Life Binary: A Feminist-Indigenous Reading of Cryopreservation, Interspecies Thinking and the New Materialisms," when I was drafting my manuscript. I sincerely thank her for her generosity. Earlier versions of this work were presented at the Society for Psychological Anthropology, the American Anthropological Association Annual Meetings, and a Suicide and Agency Workshop sponsored by the Max Planck Institute of Social Anthropology in Halle, Germany.

I am forever grateful for the formal and informal guidance I have received from various mentors over the years. At Berkeley, a dissertation committee comprised of Stanley Brandes, William Hanks, Lawrence Cohen, and William Taylor offered support during the infancy of this project. I can't think of a better team in my corner. I am especially grateful to my mentor, Stanley Brandes, who continues to be a source of wisdom and encouragement and who has always reminded me of the value of good ethnographic fieldwork. In her role as UC Berkeley department chair, Marianne Ferme provided crucial financial support at a critical moment. Laura Ahearn and Ana Yolanda Ramos-Zayas have mentored and advised me well beyond my undergraduate years at Rutgers. I am grateful for their continued friendship. Laura and Ana Yolanda both encouraged me to write this book at a time when I did not believe it would ever be written. Without them, it is very possible *Psychiatric Encounters* would have never come into being.

I am grateful to my friends and colleagues at the University of Central Florida. Sarah Stacy Barber, Sandra Wheeler, Lana Williams, Nessette Falu, Wanda Raimundi-Ortiz, Cecilia Milanés, Ilenia Colón-Mendoza, Shana Harris, Yovanna Pineda and Shannon Carter all provided moments of friendship, levity, and comfort during the writing process.

My stepfather, Professor Emeritus Alberto R. W. Green, first encouraged me to pursue anthropology and provided valuable knowledge and advice as I have navigated my career over the years. I am forever grateful for his support. My biggest cheerleader has always been my mother, Beatriz Cortes. Without her strength and fighting spirit, I would not be who I am today. Most importantly, without the solid partnership and support of my spouse, Ronald Reyes-Foster, I would never have been able to get through the excruciating demands of graduate school, three babies, and the tenure track, let alone the painstaking work of writing this book.

My children, Aydin Mateo, Rowan Salvador, and Miles Ricardo, whose arrival was awaited as of this writing, were an unknowing source of joy and inspiration.

I am indebted to the administration and psychiatrists at the facility I call Las Lomas for allowing access to the institution, for the honesty and candor with which they discussed their work, and for accepting my presence among them. Finally, it is difficult to put into words the gratitude I feel toward the patients I encountered in my time at Las Lomas. Their stories and experiences motivated me to keep moving forward with writing this book and carrying out this work even when it became emotionally difficult. I hope *Psychiatric Encounters* does their stories justice.

NOTES

1. INTRODUCTION

1. This is an interesting play on words. In Spanish, *seguro* is a word used to mean insurance, but also surety, safety, and security. The best translation I can offer to this expression is "Surety? Surely you will die!"

2. CONEVAL, Mexico's national social development policy evaluation agency, defines poverty using a multidimensional framework based on six different measures of poverty: access to education, access to health care, access to social security, quality and size of living spaces, availability of basic services (running water and electricity) in these spaces, and food security. Poverty is defined as lacking at least one of these six indicators and lacking sufficient income to gain access to them. Extreme poverty is defined by lack of access to three or more of the six indicators and an income below the "line of minimum well-being" and the "line of well-being." The "line of minimum well-being" is a variable measure based on a monthly assessment of the average cost of a "basket" of food deemed necessary for basic survival. The "line of well-being" is based on a monthly assessment of a "basket" of food plus a "basket" of nonfood items deemed necessary for daily life. In the latest figures available (2014), 52.8 percent of the population was found to be below the "line of well-being" and 20.7 percent was found to be living below the "line of minimum well-being." CONEVAL also collects information on economic vulnerability and risk of falling into poverty.

3. In this book, I use the terms "Global North" and "Global South" as designations for countries previously called "developed" and "developing," which were generally correlated to individual nation states' former status as colonizers or colonies. Mexico, because of its relatively prosperous economy and infrastructure despite its status as a former colony, challenges the boundaries of these terms. This is why I tend to think of Mexico as an example of a possible "Global Middle," because it is neither fully privileged like the wealthier Global North nor destitute like much of the Global South.

4. Writing on Brazil, DaMatta has argued that the adoption of liberal constitutions proclaiming equal rights in fact perpetuated inequalities. Gledhill (2004, 166) further argues this is because the perpetuation of corruption in Latin America is dependent on an "excessive legalism" serving the interests of the powerful (2004, 166).

5. Import Substitution Industrialization (ISI) was an economic development model premised on dependency theory, the recognition that postcolonial Latin American economies were dependent on trade relationships with wealthier "developed" nations which exploited this dependency to the poorer nations' disadvantage. Under ISI, Mexico and other countries that embraced this model invested heavily in industrialization while levying heavy tariffs on foreign goods as a way of creating sustainable, independent national economies. ISI was abandoned throughout Latin America following the economic crises of the 1980s. In Mexico, the debt crisis of 1982 made it the first of many Latin American countries to default on its sovereign debt. International Monetary Fund (IMF) and World Bank emergency funds were contingent on the abandonment of ISI in favor of incipient neoliberal economic policies. For further reading, see Shaiken (1989), Hernández Chavez (2006), and Moreno-Brid and Ros (2009).

6. This is the region where Redfield and Villa Rojas's (1934) classic, *Chan Kom: A Maya Village*, which depicts the community as highly independent and not operating in conditions of

slavery, is set (1934). However, I heard stories of esclavitud as far east as Dzipnup and Vallado-lid, two communities relatively close to Chan Kom.

7. Barenboim (2018) notes the term uuchben mako'ob can be applied to recently deceased known ancestors and/or to the builders of the pyramids. In this particular instance, I am refer-ring to the former meaning of the term.

8. *Nervios* is considered to be a culturally bound illness category used throughout Latin Amer-ica to describe various symptoms, including anxiety, panic disorder, and mood disturbances. Nervios is categorized as a "culture-bound syndrome" in the *Diagnostic and Statistical Manual of Mental Disorders of the American Psychiatric Association* (DSM-5) and the *International Sta-tistical Classification of Diseases and Related Health Problems of the World Health Organization* (ICD-10).

2. COLONIALITY, *LA ZONA DEL ESTAR*, AND YUCATAN'S MAYA HERITAGE

1. For a detailed, highly engaging analysis of Maya identity in Yucatan, see Armstrong-Fumero's (2013) monograph, *Elusive Unity: Factionalism and the Limits of Identity Politics in Yucatan, Mexico.*

2. *Pik* (Yucatec Mayan, Spanish *fustán*) is an underskirt with lace hemming worn under the huipil.

3. See Reyes-Foster (2012) for a more detailed analysis of Claudina's story. I use the word *india* here because Claudina indicated this was a word her own father used when he was being ver-bally abusive toward her.

4. *Macehual* is an Aztec class category used among the Maya territories in Yucatan at the time of contact. Archaeologists and ethnohistorians (Farriss 1985; Clendinnen 1989; Tozzer 1941; Sharer 1994) agree that Aztec and Maya social structure was highly hierarchical at the time of contact, a structure the Spanish conquistadores took advantage of in their dismantling of these societies. One could argue that the importance of class as an identity category may be, ironi-cally, indigenous.

5. I fully describe Mexico's health care schemes in Chapter 4.

6. *Chicana/o/x*, also spelled *Xicana/o/x*, generally refers to an ethnic and political identity cat-egory for people of Mexican descent born in the United States. Although its meaning is con-tested, the term is frequently discursively tied to Chicano nationalism, a movement that views Chicanos residing in the US as indigenous people occupying land that is rightfully theirs. Within this literature, Anzaldúa, alongside Sandra Cisneros, Pat Mora, Corky Gonzalez, and José Anto-nio Villareal, among others, is considered a seminal figure.

7. *Aka pacha* refers to the Andean concept of the present, which is connected to a cyclic tempo-rality unlike that of Western notions of linear time. For Rivera Cusicanqui (2010), indigenous people have a stake in their own modernity through this understanding of time understood as a constant present.

8. I did not come up with this notion myself. Karen Stolley suggested this idea in a conversa-tion during a visit to Emory University in 2017. I would like to thank Karen for making this observation and coining the term *Zona del Estar*.

9. This permanent present invites us to think about time and the present differently, much in the same way that Rivera Cusicanqui (2010) writes of aka pacha, and de Sousa Santos (2010) calls for an expansion of the present in his sociology of absence. While these also present interesting frameworks, I find the notion of Zona del Estar most useful for thinking about indigeneity and madness together. As Grosfoguel argues, there is room for epistemic plurality in decolonial think-ing. This concept is simply one way of thinking through the ethnographic material at hand.

10. The two notions—ethnoexodus and Zona del Estar—should thus be seen as different ways of understanding similar but not identical phenomena. They present two conceptual tools coexisting in epistemic plurality as kindred spirits.

11. Settler colonialism is a displacement-focused form of colonialism whereby the indigenous population is desired or expected to disappear either by relocation or death. Although it is considered global in scale, the term was originally coined to describe settlement-driven Anglo-European settlement in North America, which contrasted with Hispano-Luso settlement that sought to dominate and exploit the existing indigenous population in order to maximize the extraction of resources from the new world.

12. Obviously suicide is a complex social phenomenon. If the reader is interested in learning more about suicide in Yucatan, see Reyes-Foster (2013a, 2013b, 2014, 2016a), Reyes-Foster and Kangas (2016), and Baquedano-Lopez (2009).

13. While "heritage" for UNESCO or even for Mexico's own Instituto Nacional de Antropología e Historia (INAH) may simply refer to material culture, for anthropologists, heritage is better understood as a process (Skeates 2000) or an assemblage (Breglia 2006). This approach troubles traditional definitions of heritage that situate it within material culture and tend to conceptualize heritage as living culture that is bounded and static, hence needing "preservation."

14. The fact that Maya people themselves have taken up the mantle of Maya-ness and are now innovatively using social media to actively resist state narratives that monopolize Maya culture is a promising development, unfortunately outside of the scope of this research.

15. *Nota roja*, or red journalism, refers to a journalistic genre that focuses its attention on gore and blood. For a detailed analysis of the representation of suicides and Maya people in Yucatecan newspapers, see Reyes-Foster (2013b).

16. This trope bears some exploration, as the name "Xtabay" phonetically and linguistically approaches Ixtab. Rachael Kangas and I explore this somewhat in our 2016 article, yet a more thorough analysis is needed. It is, unfortunately, beyond the scope of this book.

3. MAKING THE MATRIX

1. Juan Vasquez, personal communication.

2. This rapport was short-lived. Dr. Tun, too, eventually had a falling out with Dr. Pasos. There was yet another change in the hospital leadership in 2015. The new director was a close personal friend of Dr. Tun. She wrote me, inviting me to return to Las Lomas. A few months later, the entire institution was rocked by a series of changes that eventually led to its administration being taken over by the federal government and by a complete turnover in its leadership. I discuss these events in the epilogue.

3. Presumably these people had enrolled prior to 2014, when automatic screening for enrollment in IMSS or ISSSTE became commonplace. Even though these dual enrollees had confirmed access to health care, the state directive was to allow them to remain enrolled until the end of their three-year policy so as to not suddenly deprive this population of medical care.

4. For further anthropological reading on corruption and society, see Gledhill (2004) and Nuijten and Anders (2007).

5. De Certeau (2002) draws an important distinction between strategies and tactics: strategies are part of the purview of power and are enacted by states and other powerful institutions. They are deliberate, planned, and operate on a large scale. Tactics are deployed by actors on the ground, based on constant assessment and reassessment of the surrounding environment. Tactics thus can be understood to exist in response—and resistance—to strategy.

6. For an excellent commentary on the anthropology of bureaucracy and anthropological approaches to bureaucracy, see Hoag (2011).

7. The institution was eventually subjected to investigation by the commission in later years (see epilogue). Moreover, Mexico's national human rights commission has been involved in efforts to address human rights violations in Mexican psychiatric institutions, even coauthoring one of Disability Rights International's reports on conditions in psychiatric institutions (DRI 2011). A case like Andrea's could have drawn their interest.

8. *Boba*: colloquial Spanish word for "dumb," "gullible," or "stupid." Doña Isabel implied that she had somehow been deceived into coming to the hospital.

9. This is merely how psychiatrists at Las Lomas interpret the nurses' behavior. As I did not have the opportunity to ask any nurses about this particular question, I cannot speak to their perspective.

4. MODERNITY

1. As of the date of this writing, Dr. Treviño continues to work at Las Lomas. He has been continuously employed at the psychiatric hospital for nearly sixty years, including his time at Las Lomas's predecessor institution. Dr. Vasquez has nearly forty years of continuous service at Las Lomas. I last saw him in August 2016, during my last visit to Las Lomas.

2. *Domingo Familiar* is the common practice in Yucatan of spending Sundays socializing with family, often involving outings to local parks and public areas such as the city zoo. Centenario is the name of the Merida city zoo.

3. For a detailed and engaging historiography of madness and psychiatry in Mexico, see Sacristán (2005).

4. The fourth federally operated health care scheme is the Military Health System.

5. In my time at Las Lomas, I never met an attending physician who did not specialize in psychiatry. Some residents were completing an integrative medicine specialization, but they were supervised by psychiatrists. I did not meet every physician employed at Las Lomas, however, so it is possible that these rumors are true.

6. *Acordión* literally translates to "accordion," yet the word is also used to signify a commonly used cheating technique whereby exam answers are written on a sheet of paper folded like an accordion. *Acordiones* are a fixture in Mexican grade schools.

7. This admonishment to respect is evocative of Castillo Cocom's (2005; Castillo Cocom and Ríos Luviano 2012) argument that politics in Yucatan is marked by a lack of respect for indigenous people, particularly as local political parties attempt to subsume them by recognizing specific allies as indigenous leaders over others.

8. The bilingual signage throughout the hospital is a recent addition, appearing in the wake of a human rights investigation that took place after I left the field (see the epilogue).

9. Literally "son" in Spanish, commonly used as a term of endearment between spouses.

5. NEGOTIATING TRUTH IN THE PSYCHIATRIC ENCOUNTER

1. Eva's case is further analyzed in chapter 6.

2. Part of the goal of the clinical session for psychiatric residents is to hone their diagnostic skills. The axes discussed in this session refer to the DSM-4 multiaxial diagnostic system, which assigns an axis to particular domains of human experience. Broadly speaking, Axis I refers to clinical disorders, Axis II to personality disorders, Axis III to medical or physical disorders, Axis IV to environmental or social effects. Finally, Axis V is the Global Assessment of Functioning (GAF) score, a 100-point scale that measures functionality and ability to engage in daily life. Although the DSM-5 moved away from the multiaxial diagnosis system, in 2012 the DSM-5 had not yet been published, and DSM-4 was still the most commonly used diagnostic guide in training psychiatric residents in Mexico, despite the fact that the official diagnostic manual of Las Lomas was the WHO's ICD-10 guide, which also has a multiaxial diagnosis formulation, albeit one that is different from that of the DSM-4.

3. After I concluded my field research inside Las Lomas in 2012, the hospital was subjected to repeated criticism in the local news media. Accusations of human rights violations were leveraged, and improvements to the facilities were made following supervision from the local Commission for the Protection of Human Rights. I discuss these events further in the epilogue.

4. The equivalent of a U.S. bachelor's degree.

5. Manuela's diagnosis when I last saw her was ICD-10 diagnosis F23, Schizophreniform Brief Psychotic Disorder. She was still committed to Las Lomas, but was considered to have made significant progress, when my time there ended.

6. As I discussed in Chapter 4, this—alongside with the worrying report that he was refusing food—may be what prompted her to suggest to Don Gustavo's family that they "double up" on health insurance to get access to Seguro Popular's medications.

7. For an interesting account of practitioner promises and misfirings when these promises fall flat, see Chua (2012).

6. IN THE HEART OF MADNESS

1. Of course, Mauss argued about the inalienability of the gift long before Strathern.

2. Latour refers to these beings as the "Beings of Metamorphosis" in his description of [met] as a mode of existence (2013, 194). I engage more thoroughly with Latour's arguments in *An Inquiry into Modes of Existence* in Reyes-Foster (2016b).

3. Lucas Bessire and David Bond make this argument very compellingly, focusing on what they consider Amerindian Perspectivism's collapse of the nature/culture binary in Bessire (2014), Bessire and Bond (2014), and Bond and Bessire (2014).

4. I explore Claudina's story in Reyes-Foster (2012).

5. Juan always said that suicide attempts were not *intentos de muerte* (attempts to die), but *intentos de vida* (attempts to live).

6. My dissertation was ultimately titled "Adoring Our Wounds."

7. Panuchos are a popular Yucatecan dish. They consist of a deep-fried corn tortilla filled with refried black beans, topped with chicken, lettuce, and tomato. Many people in Mexico supplement their income by making and selling panuchos out of their homes.

8. Although this version of the turn is particularly relevant to this chapter, his critique does not resonate as deeply with the bodily ontology of Annemarie Mol (2003), the relational ontology of Marilyn Strathern (2005), the new materialisms of Jane Bennett (2010 and Mel Chen (2012), or Latour's own writings (2007, 2013) on objects with agency and invisible beings as they pertain to actor-network theory and modes of existence.

7. EPILOGUE

1. Although I have tried to disguise key details about my interlocutors, it would not be difficult for someone very familiar with Las Lomas to deduce their identities. For this reason, I am being deliberately coy about the individual opinions held by any of my interlocutors about recent events. Thanks to contemporary communication technologies, I maintain ties with

nearly all the hospital staff I encountered in my time at Las Lomas, and some former patients. I am also omitting specific citations to local news coverage of events.

2. Some may argue that the history of mental institutions goes further back to the original founding of Hospital San Hipólito by Bernardino Álvarez in 1560 (Fernández del Castillo 1966). However, I follow historian Cristina Sacristán's suggestion that this represents more of hagiography than a history of psychiatry in Mexico. San Hipólito did not begin to function as a mental asylum in the modern sense until the mid-nineteenth century, and it was replaced by the manicomio La Castañeda in 1910, during the Porfiriato.

BIBLIOGRAPHY

Abu-Lughod, Lila. 1991. "Writing against Culture." In *Recapturing Anthropology: Working in the Present*, edited by Richard G. Fox, 137–154. Santa Fe, NM: School of American Research Press.

Agamben, Giorgio. 1995. *Homo Sacer: Sovereign Power and Bare Life*. Stanford, CA: Stanford University Press.

Almaguer González, J., V. Vargas Vite, and H. J. García Ramírez. 2014. *Interculturalidad en Salud: Experiencias y Aportes para el Fortalecimiento de los Servicios de Salud*. Mexico City: Gobierno de la República.

American Psychiatric Association. 2013. *Diagnostic and Statistical Manual of Mental Disorders (DSM-5)*. Arlington, VA: American Psychiatric Association.

Anzaldúa, Gloria. 1987. *Borderlands/La Frontera: The New Mestiza*. San Francisco: Aunt Lute Books.

Appadurai, Arjun. 1996. *Modernity at Large: Cultural Dimensions of Globalization*. Minneapolis: University of Minnesota Press.

Armstrong-Fumero, Fernando. 2009. "A Heritage of Ambiguity: The Historical Substrate of Vernacular Multiculturalism in Yucatán, Mexico." *American Ethnologist* 36 (2): 300–316.

Armstrong-Fumero, Fernando. 2013. *Elusive Unity: Factionalism and the Limits of Identity Politics in Yucatan, Mexico*. Boulder: University Press of Colorado.

Arndt, Grant. 2016. "Settler Agnosia in the Field: Indigenous Action, Functional Ignorance, and the Origins of Ethnographic Entrapment." *American Ethnologist* 43 (3): 465–474.

Baquedano-Lopez, Gaspar. 2009. "Maya Religion and Traditions: Influencing Suicide Prevention in Contemporary Mexico." In *Oxford Textbook of Suicidology and Suicide Prevention: A Global Perspective*, edited by D. Wasserman and C. Wasserman, 77–84. New York: Oxford University Press.

Barenboim, Deanna. 2018. "Reclaiming Tangible Heritage: Cultural Aesthetics, Materiality, and Ethnic Belonging in the Maya Diaspora." *Journal of Latin American and Caribbean Anthropology* (forthcoming).

Barry, Andrew, Thomas Osborne, and Nikolas Rose. 1996. *Foucault and Political Reason: Liberalism, Neo-liberalism, and Rationalities of Government*. Chicago: University of Chicago Press.

Bennett, Jane. 2010. *Vibrant Matter: A Political Ecology of Things*. Durham, NC: Duke University Press.

Bessire, Lucas. 2014. *Behold the Black Caiman: A Chronicle of Ayoreo Life*. Chicago: University of Chicago Press.

Bessire, Lucas, and David Bond. 2014. "Ontological Anthropology and the Deferral of Critique." *American Ethnologist* 41 (3): 440–456.

Bhabha, Homi. 2004. "Foreword: Framing Fanon." In *The Wretched of the Earth*, by Frantz Fanon. Translated by Richard Philcox. New York: Grove Press.

Biehl, João. 2005. *Vita: Life in a Zone of Social Abandonment*. Berkeley: University of California Press.

Biehl, João, Byron Good, and Arthur Kleinman, eds. 2007. *Subjectivity: Ethnographic Investigations*. Berkeley: University of California Press.

Blagg, Harry. 2016. "From Terra Nullius to Terra Liquidus? Liquid Modernity and the Indigenous Other." In *Punishing the Other: The Social Production of Immorality Revisited*, edited by Anna Erikson. New York: Routledge.

Boffil Gómez, Luis. 2008. "Para labores personal de 18 hospitales de Mérida; rechazan imposición de director." *La Jornada*, May 17.

Bond, David, and Lucas Bessire. 2014. "The Ontological Spin." *Cultural Anthropology*, February 28, 2014. https://culanth.org/fieldsights/494-the-ontological-spin.

Bonfil Batalla, Guillermo. 1987. *El México Profundo: Una Civilización Negada*. Mexico City: Editorial Grijalbo.

Breglia, Lisa. 2006. *Monumental Ambivalence: The Politics of Heritage*. Austin: University of Texas Press.

Briggs, Charles, and Richard Bauman. 1999. "'The Foundation of All Future Researches': Franz Boas, Native American Texts, and the Construction of Modernity." *American Quarterly* 51 (3): 479–528.

Butler, Judith. (1990) 1999. *Gender Trouble*. New York: Routledge.

Calderón Narváez, G. 1996a. "La Psiquiatría en México: Principios del Siglo XX (1900–1950)." *Archivo de Neurociencias* 1 (1): 27–34.

———. 1996b. "La Psiquiatría en México: Década de los Cincuenta y Principios de los Sesenta (1950–1965)." *Archivo de Neurociencias* 1 (4): 303–310.

———. 2002. *Las Enfermedades Mentales en México: Desde los Mexicas hasta el Final del Milenio*. Mexico City: Editorial Trillas.

Carlson, John B. 2011. "Anticipating the Maya Apocalypse: What Might the Ancient Day-Keepers Have Envisioned for December 21, 2012?" *Archaeoastronomy* 24:143–182.

Carr, E. Summerson. 2011. *Scripting Addiction: The Politics of Therapeutic Talk and American Sobriety*. Princeton, NJ: Princeton University Press.

Carrithers, Michael, Matei Candea, Karen Sykes, Martin Holbraad, and Soumhya Venkatesan. 2010. "Ontology Is Just Another Word for Culture: Motion Tabled at the 2008 Meeting of the Group for Debates in Anthropological Theory, University of Manchester." *Critique of Anthropology* 30 (2): 152–200.

Castañeda, Quetzil. 1996. *In the Museum of Maya Culture: Touring Chichén Itzá*. Minneapolis: University of Minnesota Press.

———. 2004. "'We Are Not Indigenous!': An Introduction to the Maya Identity of Yucatan." *Journal of Latin American and Caribbean Anthropology* 9 (1): 36–63.

Castillo Cocom, Juan. 2005. "'It Was Simply Their Word': Yucatec Maya PRInces in YucaPAN and the Politics of Respect." *Critique of Anthropology* 25 (2): 131–155.

Castillo Cocom, Juan, and Saúl Ríos Luviano. 2012. "Hot and Cold Politics of Indigenous Identity: Legal Indians, Cannibals, Words, More Words, More Food." *Anthropological Quarterly* 85 (1): 229–256.

Castillo Cocom, Juan, Timoteo Rodriguez, and McCale Ashenbrender. 2017. "Ethnoexodus: Escaping Mayaland." In *"The Only True People": Linking Maya Identities Past and Present*, edited by Bethany Beyyette and Lisa LeCount, 47–72. Boulder: University Press of Colorado.

Cha'anil Kaaj. 2015. "Cha'anil Kaaj: Fiesta Propositiva de Difusión y Libre Expresión de las Manifestaciones Culturales y Sociales del Pueblo." (Cha'anil Kaaj official website) http://www.chaanilkaaj.org/index.html.

Chen, Mel. 2012. *Animacies: Biopolitics, Racial Mattering, and Queer Affect*. Durham, NC: Duke University Press.

Chua, Jocelyn. 2012. "The Register of Complaint: Psychiatric Diagnosis and the Discourse of Grievance in the South Indian Mental Health Encounter." *Medical Anthropology Quarterly* 26 (2): 221–240.

Clendinnen, Inga. 1989. *Ambivalent Conquests: Maya and Spaniard in Yucatan, 1517–1570*. Cambridge: Cambridge University Press.

Consejo Nacional de Evaluación de la Política de Desarrollo Social (CONEVAL). 2014. *Informe de Pobreza en México, 2014.* Mexico City: CONEVAL.

Coole, Diana, and Samatha Frost, eds. 2010. *New Materialisms: Ontology, Agency, and Politics.* Durham, NC: Duke University Press.

Correll, Christoph, Christine Rummel-Kluge, Caroline Corves, John M. Kane, and Stefan Leucht. 2009. "Antipsychotic Combinations vs. Monotherapy in Schizophrenia: A Meta-analysis of Randomized Controlled Trials." *Schizophrenia Bulletin: Journal of Psychoses and Related Disorders* 35 (2): 443–457.

Das, Jishnu, Quy-Toan Do, Jed Friedman, David McKenzie, and Kinnon Scott. 2007. "Mental Health and Poverty in Developing Countries: Revisiting the Relationship." *Social Science & Medicine* 65 (3): 467–480.

Davis, Elizabeth. 2010. "The Antisocial Profile: Deception and Intimacy in Greek Psychiatry." *Cultural Anthropology* 25 (1): 130–164.

———. 2012. *Bad Souls: Madness and Responsibility in Modern Greece.* Durham, NC: Duke University Press.

de Certeau, Michel. 2002. *The Practice of Everyday Life.* Berkeley: University of California Press.

de Rodrigo, Enrique. 2015. *Neoliberalismo y Otras Patologías de la Normalidad: Conversando Nuestro Tiempo con Erich Fromm.* Madrid: PenBooks.

Deloria, Vine Jr. 2001. "American Indian Metaphysicis." In *Power and Place: Indian Education in America,* edited by Vine Deloria Jr. and Daniel Wildcat, 1–6. Golden, CO: Fulcrum Publishing.

Descola, Philippe. 2013. *Beyond Nature and Culture.* Translated by Janet Lloyd. Chicago: University of Chicago Press, 2013.

de Silva, Denise Ferreira. 2007. *Toward a Global Idea of Race.* Minneapolis: University of Minnesota Press.

de Sousa Santos, Boaventura. 2010. *Descolonizar el Saber, Reinventar el Poder.* Montevideo, Uruguay: Ediciones Trilce.

Diario de Yucatán. 2016. "Indigentes del centro de Mérida, con familia que no los atiende." Saturday, May 21. http://yucatan.com.mx/merida/ciudadanos/indigentes-del-centro-de-merida-con-familia-que-no-los-atiende.

———. 2017. "Realidad con muchas caras: Aumentan casos de menesterosos con discapacidad." Saturday, August 19. http://yucatan.com.mx/merida/realidad-muchas-caras.

Diocaretz, Myriam, and Stefan Herbrechter. 2006. *The Matrix in Theory.* New York: Rodopi.

Disability Rights International (DRI). 2011. *Abandoned & Disappeared: Mexico's Segregation and Abuse of Children and Adults with Disabilities.* Washington, DC: Disability Rights International & Comisión Nacional de Defensa y Promoción de los Derechos Humanos.

———. 2015. *No Justice: Torture, Trafficking and Segregation in Mexico.* Washington, DC: Disability Rights International.

Duncan, Whitney. 2017. "*Psicoeducación* in the Land of Magical Thinking: Culture and Mental-Health Practice in a Changing Oaxaca." *American Ethnologist* 44 (1): 1–16.

Echeverría, Bolívar. 2010. *Modernidad y Blanquitud.* Mexico City: Era.

Emmerich, Roland, dir. 2009. *2012.* Culver City, CA: Sony Pictures.

Engels, Frederick. 1993. *The Condition of the Working Class in England.* Oxford: Oxford University Press.

Fallaw, Ben. 2001. *Cárdenas Compromised: The Failure of Reform in Postrevolutionary Yucatán.* Durham, NC: Duke University Press.

Fanon, Frantz. (1952) 2008. *Black Skin, White Masks.* Translated by Richard Philcox. New York: Grove.

————. (1961) 2004. *The Wretched of the Earth*. Translated by Richard Philcox. New York: Grove Press.

Farmer, Paul. 2004. *Pathologies of Power: Health, Human Rights, and the New War on the Poor*. Berkeley: University of California Press.

Farriss, Nancy. 1985. *Maya Society under Colonial Rule: The Collective Enterprise of Survival*. Princeton, NJ: Princeton University Press.

Ferguson, James, and Akhil Gupta. 2002. "Spatializing States: Towards an Ethnography of Neoliberal Governmentality." *American Ethnologist* 29 (4): 981–1002.

Fernández del Castillo, Francisco. 1966. "Bernardino Alvarez, Iniciador de la atención neuropsiquiátrica en México (1566–1966)." *Gaceta Médica de México* 96 (9): 1013–1022.

Forman, Miloš, dir. 1975. *One Flew Over the Cuckoo's Nest*. United Artists.

Foucault, Michel. 1972. *Power/Knowledge: Selected Interviews and Other Writings*. Translated by C. Gordon. New York: Random House.

————. 1988a. *Madness and Civilization: A History of Insanity in the Age of Reason*. Translated by Richard Howard. New York: Vintage Books. Original edition 1965.

————. 1988b. Confinement, Psychiatry, Prison. In *Michel Foucault: Politics Philosophy Culture*, edited by L. D. Kritzman, 178–210. New York: Routledge.

Fromm, Erich. 1990. *Man for Himself: An Inquiry into the Psychology of Ethics*. New York: Holt.

Funk, Rainer. 2003. *Erich Fromm: His Life and Ideas*. Translated by I. Portman and M. Kunkel. New York: Continuum International Publishing Group.

Gamio, Manuel. 2010. *Forjando Patria (Forging a Nation)*. Translated by Fernando Armstrong-Fumero. Boulder: University of Colorado Press.

García Canclini, Nestor. 1989. *Culturas Híbridas: Estrategias para Entrar y Salir de la Modernidad*. Mexico City: Grijalbo, CONACULTA.

————. 2005. "Introduction: Hybrid Cultures in Globalized Times." In *Hybrid Cultures: Strategies for Entering and Leaving Modernity*, xxiii–xlvi. Minneapolis: University of Minnesota Press.

Gledhill, John. 2004. "Corruption as the Mirror of the State in Latin America." In *Between Morality and the Law: Corruption, Anthropology and Comparative Society*, edited by Italo Pardo, 155–180. Burlington, VT: Ashgate.

Gobierno de la República. 2013. *Plan Nacional de Desarrollo, 2013–2018: Programa Sectorial de Salud*. Mexico City: Gobierno de la República.

Gone, Joseph. 2014. "Colonial Genocide and Historical Trauma in Native North America: Complicating Contemporary Attributions." In *Colonial Genocide in Indigenous North America*, edited by Andrew Woolford, Jeff Benvenuto, and Alexander Laban Hinton. Durham, NC: Duke University Press.

González Casanova, Pedro. 1969. *Sociología de la Explotación*. Mexico City: Grijalbo.

Good, Byron. 1997. "Studying Mental Illness in Context: Local, Global, or Universal." *Ethos* 25 (2): 230–248.

Graeber, David. 2015. "Radical Alterity Is Just Another Way of Saying 'Reality': A Reply to Eduartdo Viveiros de Castro." *Hau Journal of Ethnographic Theory* 5 (2): 1–41.

Greensmith, Cameron. 2012. "Pathologizing Indigeneity in the Caledonia 'Crisis.'" *Canadian Journal of Disability Studies* 1 (2): 19–42.

Grosfoguel, Ramón. 2011a. "Decolonizing Post-Colonial Studies and Paradigms of Political-Economy: Transmodernity, Decolonial Thinking, and Global Coloniality." *Transmodernity: Journal of the Peripheral Cultural Production of the Luso-Hispanic World* 1 (1). https://escholarship.org/uc/item/21k6t3fq.

————. 2011b. "La Descolonización del Conocimiento: Diálogo Crítico entre la Visión Descolonial de Frantz Fanon y la Sociología Descolonial de Boaventura de Sousa Santos."

In *Formas-Otras: Saber, Nombrar, Narar, Hacer*, edited by Boaventura de Sousa Santos, 97–108. Barcelona: CIDOB Ediciones.

Guarnaccia, Peter, Victor DeLaCancela, and Emilio Carrillo. 1989. "The Multiple Meanings of Ataques de Nervios in the Latino Community." *Medical Anthropology: Cross Cultural Studies in Health and Illness* 11 (1): 47–62.

Guarnaccia, Peter, Melissa Rivera, Felipe Franco, and Charlie Neighbors. 1996. "The Experiences of Ataques de Nervios: Towards an Anthropology of Emotions in Puerto Rico." *Culture, Medicine and Psychiatry* 20 (3): 343–367.

Gupta, Akhil. 1995. "Blurred Boundaries: The Discourse of Corruption, the Culture of Politics, and the Imagined State." *American Ethnologist* 22 (2): 375–402.

Hanks, William F. 1990. *Referential Practice: Language and Lived Space among the Maya*. Chicago: University of Chicago Press.

Hayden, Cori. 2007. "A Generic Solution? Pharmaceuticals and the Politics of the Similar in Mexico." *Current Anthropology* 48 (4): 475–495.

HealthGrove. 2013. "Schizophrenia in Mexico: Statistics on Overall Impact and Specific Effect on Demographic Groups." Accessed February 13. http://global-disease-burden.healthgrove.com/l/58163/Schizophrenia-in-Mexico - References&s=ref.

Hernández Chavez, Alicia. 2006. *Mexico: A Brief History*. Berkeley: University of California Press.

Hervik, Peter. 2003. *Mayan People within and beyond Boundaries: Social Categories and Lived Identity in the Yucatan*. New York: Routledge.

Hirose, Javier. 2008. "El ser humano como eje cósmico: las concepciones del cuerpo y la persona entre los mayas de la region de los chenes, Campeche." PhD, Estudios Mesoamericanos, Universidad Nacional Autónoma de México.

Hoag, Colin. 2011. "Assembling Partial Perspectives: Thoughts on the Anthropology of Bureaucracy." *PoLAR: Political and Legal Anthropology Review* 34 (1): 81–94.

Homedes, Núria, and Antonio Ugalde. (2009). Twenty-Five Years of Convoluted Health Reforms in Mexico. *PLoS Medicine* 6 (8): e1000124.

Horcasitas, Urías. 2000. *Indígena y Criminal: Interpretaciones del Derecho y la Antropología en México, 1871–1921*. Mexico City: Universidad Iberoamericana.

Hughes, Karen, Mark Bellis, Lisa Jones, Sara Wood, Geoff Bates, Lindsay Eckley, Ellie McCoy, Christopher Mikton, Tom Shakespeare, and Alana Officer. 2012. "Prevalence and Risk of Violence against Adults with Disabilities: A Systematic Review and Meta-analysis of Observational Studies." *Lancet* 380 (9845): 899–907.

Illouz, E. 2008. *Saving the Modern Soul: Therapy, Emotions, and the Culture of Self-Help*. Berkeley: University of California Press.

Instituto Nacional De Estadística, Geografía, e Informática (INEGI). 2016. Derechohabiencia y Uso de Servicios de Salud. Mexico: INEGI.

Jenkins, Janis. 2015. *Extraordinary Conditions: Culture and Experience in Mental Illness*. Berkeley: University of California Press.

Joseph, Gilbert. 2010. "Some Final Thoughts on Regional History and the Encounter with Modernity at Mexico's Periphery." In *Peripheral Visions: Politics, Society, and the Challenges of Modernity of Yucatan*, edited by Edward Terry, Ben Fallaw, Gilbert Joseph, and Edward H. Moseley, 254–266. Tuscaloosa: University of Alabama Press.

Kleinman, Arthur. 1980. *Patients and Healers in the Context of Culture: An Exploration of the Borderland between Anthropology, Medicine, and Psychiatry*. Berkeley: University of California Press.

Kral, Michael. 2012. "Postcolonial Suicide among Inuit in Arctic Canada." *Culture, Medicine and Psychiatry* 36 (2): 326.

Lakoff, Andrew. 2005. *Pharmaceutical Reason: Knowledge and Value in Global Psychiatry.* Cambridge: Cambridge University Press.

Latour, Bruno. 2007. *Reassembling the Social: An Introduction to Actor-Network Theory.* Oxford: Oxford University Press.

———. 2013. *An Inquiry into Modes of Existence: An Anthropology of the Moderns.* Cambridge, MA: Harvard University Press.

Leshem, Noam. 2017. "Spaces of Abandonment: Genealogies, Lives, and Critical Horizons." *Environment and Planning D: Society and Space* 35 (4): 620–636.

Levy-Orlick, Noemi. 2009. "Protectionism and Industrialization: A Critical Assessment of the Latin American Industrialization Period." *Brazilian Journal of Political Economy* 29 (4): 436–453.

Llamas, Ana, and Susan Mayhew. 2016. "The Emergence of the Vertical Birth in Ecuador: An Analysis of Agenda Setting and Policy Windows for Intercultural Health." *Health Policy and Planning* 31 (6): 683–690.

Lucas d'Oliveira, Ana, Simone Grilo Diniz, and Lilia Schraiber. 2002. "Violence against Women in Health Care Institutions: An Emerging Problem." *Lancet* 359 (9318): 1681–1685.

Luhrmann, Tanya. 2000. *Of Two Minds: An Anthropologist Looks at American Psychiatry.* New York: Vintage Books.

———. 2016. "Introduction." In *Our Most Troubling Madness: Case Studies in Schizophrenia across Cultures,* edited by Tanya Luhrmann and Jocelyn Marrow, 1–26. Berkeley: University of California Press.

Luhrmann, Tanya, and Jocelyn Marrow. 2016. *Our Most Troubling Madness: Case Studies in Schizophrenia across Cultures.* Berkeley: University of California Press.

Lund, Crick, Mary De Silva, Sophie Plagerson, Sara Cooper, Dan Chisholm, Jishnu Das, Martin Knapp, and Vikram Patel. 2011. "Poverty and Mental Disorders: Breaking the Cycle in Low-Income and Middle-Income Countries." *Lancet* 378 (9801): 1502–1514.

Marín, Guillermo. 2001. *La Corrupción en Mexico: Una estrategia de resistencia cultural.* Oaxaca, Mexico: Instituto Luis Sarmiento.

Marrow, Jocelyn, and Tanya Luhrmann. 2012. "The Zone of Social Abandonment in Cultural Geography: On the Street in the United States, Inside the Family in India." *Culture, Medicine, and Psychiatry* 36 (3): 493–513.

Martineau, Jarrett. 2014. "Pat Boy: Mayan Rap Is Bringing the Culture Back." *Indigenous Music Culture.* October 1. http://rpm.fm/news/pat-boy-revitalize-mayan-culture-hip-hop/.

Martínez Novo, Carmen. 2003. "The 'Culture' of Exclusion: Representations of Indigenous Women Street Vendors in Tijuana, Mexico." *Bulletin of Latin American Research* 22 (3): 249–268.

Mayer-Serra, Carlos Elizondo. 2014. "La cultura de la corrupción." *Excelsior,* August 28. http://www.excelsior.com.mx/opinion/carlos-elizondo-mayer-serra/2014/08/28/978645.

Mental Disability Rights International (MDRI). 2000. *Human Rights and Mental Health in Mexico.* Washington, DC: Mental Disability Rights International.

Mignolo, Walter. 2000. *Local Histories/Global Designs: Coloniality, Subaltern Knowledges, and Border Thinking.* Princeton, NJ: Princeton University Press.

———. 2003. *The Darker Side of the Renaissance: Literacy, Territoriality, and Colonization,* 2nd ed. Ann Arbor: University of Michigan Press.

———. 2011. *The Darker Side of Western Modernity: Global Futures, Decolonial Options.* Durham, NC: Duke University Press.

Mol, Annemarie. 2003. *The Body Multiple: Ontology in Medical Practice, Science and Cultural Theory.* Durham, NC: Duke University Press.

Moreno-Brid, Juan Carlos, and Jaime Ros. 2009. *Development and Growth in the Mexican Economy.* Oxford: Oxford University Press.

Morris, Stephen. 1991. *Corruption and Politics in Contemporary Mexico.* Tuscaloosa: University of Alabama Press.

———. 2009. *Political Corruption in Mexico: The Impact of Democratization.* Boulder, CO: Lynne Rienner Publishers.

———. 2011. "Mexico's Political Culture: The Unrule of Law and Corruption as a Form of Resistance." *Mexican Law Review* 3 (1): 327–342.

Moseley, Edward H., and Edward Terry. 1980. *Yucatan: A World Apart.* Tuscaloosa: University of Alabama Press.

NASA. 2012. "Beyond 2012: Why the World Didn't End." In *Why the World Didn't End Yesterday,* edited by NASA Administration. NASA. https://www.nasa.gov/topics/earth/features /2012.html.

Nieto, Nubia. 2013. "La corrupción política en México: del pasado a la transición democrática." *OBETS. Revista de Ciencias Sociales* 18 (1): 127–145.

Nuijten, Monique. 2003. *Power, Community and the State: The Political Anthropology of Organisation in Mexico.* Sterling, VA: Pluto Press.

Nuijten, Monique, and Gerhard Anders. 2007. *Corruption and the Secret of Law: A Legal Anthropological Perspective.* Burlington, VT: Ashgate Press.

Paz, Octavio. (1950) 1993. *El laberinto de la Soledad, Postdata, Vuelta a "El laberinto de la soledad."* Mexico City: Fondo de la Cultura Económica.

Petrides, Georgios, Max Fink, Mustafa Husain, Rebecca Knapp, A. John Rush, Martina Mueller, Teresa Rummans, Kevin O'Conner, Keith Rasmussen, Hilary Bernstein, Melanie Biggs, Samuel Bailine, and Charles Kellner. 2001. "ECT Remission Rates in Psychotic versus Nonpsychotic Depressed Patients: A Report from GORE." *Journal of ECT* 17 (4): 244–253.

Priego, Natalia. 2012. "Porfirio Díaz, Positivism and 'The Scientists': A Reconsideration of the Myth." *Journal of Iberian and Latin American Research* 18 (2): 135–150.

Proceso. 2008. "Yucatán: Trabajadores del sector salud se suman al paro del Hospital de Alta Especialidad." *Proceso,* May 17.

Quijano, Aníbal. 1992. "Colonialidad y Modernidad/racionalidad." In *Los Conquistados: 1492 y la Población Indígena de América,* edited by Heraclio Bonilla, 437–447. Bogotá: Tercer Mundo/FLACSO.

———. 2000. "Coloniality of Power, Ethnocentrism, and Latin America." *Nepantla* 1 (3): 533–580.

Ramos, Jorge. 2015. "Ya Chole con la Corrupción." *Reforma,* October 24, 2015, Opinion. http:// www.reforma.com/aplicacioneslibre/preacceso/articulo/default.aspx?__rval=1&id =74286&urlredirect=http://www.reforma.com/aplicaciones/editoriales/editorial.aspx ?id=74286.

Re Cruz, Alicia. 1996. *The Two Milpas of Chan Kom: A Study of Socioeconomic and Political Transformations in a Maya Community.* Albany: State University of New York.

Redfield, Robert, and Alfonso Villa Rojas. 1934. *Chan Kom: A Maya Village.* Washington, DC: Carnegie Institution of Washington.

Restall, Matthew, and Amara Solari. 2011. *2012 and the End of the World: The Western Roots of the Maya Apocalypse.* Lanham, MD: Rowman and Littlefield.

Reyes Heroles, Federico. 2001. *Corrupción: De los ángeles a los índices.* Edited by Arturo del Castillo, Mauricio Merino, and Pedro Salazar. Vol. 1 of *Cuadernos de Transparencia.* Mexico City: Instituto Federal de Acceso a la Información Pública (IFAI).

———. 2015. "La Factura." *Excelsior,* September 22, 2015, Opinion.

Reyes-Foster, Beatriz. 2012. "Grieving for Mestizaje: Alternative Approaches to Maya Identity in Yucatan, Mexico." *Identities*, 1–16. https://doi.org/10.1080/1070289x.2012.734766.

———. 2013a. "The Devil Made Her Do It: Understanding Suicide, Demonic Discourse, and the Social Construction of 'Health' in Yucatan, Mexico." *Religion and Violence* 1 (3): 1–20.

———. 2013b. "He Followed the Funereal Steps of Ixtab: The Pleasurable Aesthetics of Suicide in Newspaper Journalism in Yucatán, Mexico." *Journal of Latin American and Caribbean Anthropology* 18 (2): 251–273. https://doi.org/10.1111/jlca.12019.

———. 2014. "Creating Order in the Bureaucratic Register: An Analysis of Suicide Crime Scene Investigations in Southern Mexico." *Critical Discourse Studies* 11 (4): 377–396.

———. 2016a. "Between Demons and Disease: Suicide and Agency in Yucatan, Mexico." In *Suicide and Agency: Anthropological Perspectives on Self-Destruction, Personhood, and Power*, edited by Daniel Müenster and Ludek Broz, 67–84. Burlington, VT: Ashgate Press.

———. 2016b. "Latour's AIME, Indigenous Critique, and Ontological Turns in a Mexican Psychiatric Hospital: Approaching Registers of Visibility in Three Conceptual Turns." *Anthropological Quarterly* 89 (4): 1175–1200.

Reyes-Foster, Beatriz, and Rachael Kangas. 2016. "Unraveling Ix Tab: Revisiting the Ancient Maya Suicide Goddess in Archaeology." *Ethnohistory* 63 (1): 1–27.

Ríos, Gabriela. 2016. "Mestizaje." In *Decolonizing Rhetoric and Composition: Latinx Keywords*, edited by Iris D. Ruiz and Raúl Sánchez, 109–124. New York: Springer.

Ríos Molina, Andrés. 2009. *La Locura Durante la Revolución Mexicana: Los Primeros Años del Manicomio General La Castañeda, 1910–1920*. Mexico: El Colegio de México.

Rivera Cusicanqui, Silvia. 2010. *Ch'ixinakax Utxiwa: Una Reflexión sobre las Prácticas y Discursos Descolonizadores*. Buenos Aires: Tinta Limón.

———. 2012. "Ch'ixinakax utxiwa: A Reflection on the Practices and Discourses of Decolonization." *South Atlantic Article* 111 (1): 95–109.

Rivkin-Fish, Michele. 2005. *Women's Health in Post-Soviet Russia: The Politics of Intervention*. Bloomington: Indiana University Press.

Roach, John. 2011. "End of World in 2012? Maya 'Doomsday' Calendar Explained." *National Geographic News*, December 20. https://news.nationalgeographic.com/news/2011/12/111220-end-of-world-2012-maya-calendar-explained-ancient-science/.

Rodriguez, Timoteo, and Juan Castillo Cocom. 2010. "Iknal, Identity Politics and Decolonizing the Ethnos: Yucatec Maya Epistemology." *Patrimonialisations: enjeux identitaires et problèmatiques de dèveloppement*. Paris.

Rose, Nikolas. 1996. *Inventing Our Selves: Psychology, Power, and Personhood*. Cambridge: Cambridge University Press.

Rubí, Mauricio. 2014. "Corrupción en México, un problema cultural: Peña Nieto." *El Economista*, September 8.

Sacristán, Cristina. 2005. "Historiografía de la Locura y de la Psiquiatría en México: De la Hagiografía a la Historia Posmoderna." *Frenia: Revista de Historia de la Psiquiatría* 5 (1): 9–33.

Salinas, Abigail. 2016. "Tiene Seguro Popular 82 mil Derechohabientes con IMSS e ISSSTE." *EL Diario NTR*, January 24. http://ntrzacatecas.com/2016/01/24/tiene-seguro-popular-82-mil-derechohabientes-con-imss-e-issste/.

Sánchez de Aguilar, Pedro. (1639) 2003. *Informe Contra Idolorum Cultores del Obispado de Yucatán*. Biblioteca Virtual Miguel de Cervantes.

Scheper-Hughes, Nancy. 1985. "Culture, Scarcity, and Maternal Thinking: Maternal Detachment and Infant Survival in a Brazilian Shantytown." *Ethos* 13 (4): 291–317.

Scott, James C. 1985. *Weapons of the Weak: Everyday Forms of Peasant Resistance*. New Haven, CT: Yale University Press.

Secretaría de Salud. 2007. *Programa Sectorial de Salud 2007–2012*. Mexico City: Secretaría de Salud.

Shaiken, Harley. 1989. *Mexico in the Global Economy: High Technology and Work Organization in Export Industries*. San Diego: Center for U.S.-Mexican Studies.

Sharer, Robert. 1994. *The Ancient Maya*, 5th ed. Palo Alto, CA: Stanford University Press.

Shorter, Edward, and David Healy. 2012. *Shock Therapy: A History of Electroconvulsive Treatment in Mental Illness*. New Brunswick, NJ: Rutgers University Press.

Simpson, Audra. 2007. "On Ethnographic Refusal: Indigeneity, 'Voice' and Colonial Citizenship." *Junctures: Journal for Thematic Dialogue* 9:67–80.

———. 2014. *Mohawk Interruptus*. Durham, NC: Duke University Press.

Simpson, Sharleen. 1988. "Some Preliminary Considerations on the Sobada: A Traditional Treatment for Gastrointestinal Illness in Costa Rica." *Social Science & Medicine* 27 (1): 69–73.

Skeates, Robin. 2000. *Debating the Archaeological Heritage*. London: Duckworth.

Smith, Andrea. 2014. "Native Studies at the Horizon of Death: Theorizing Ethnographic Entrapment and Settler Self-Reflexivity." In *Theorizing Native Studies*, edited by Andrea Smith and Audra Simpson. Durham, NC: Duke University Press.

Smith, Daniel. 2007. *A Culture of Corruption: Everyday Deception and Popular Discontent in Nigeria*. Princeton, NJ: Princeton University Press.

Smith-Oka, Vannia. 2013. *Shaping the Motherhood of Indigenous Mexico*. Nashville, TN: Vanderbilt University Press.

Stevenson, Lisa. 2014. *Life Beside Itself: Imagining Care in the Canadian Arctic*. Berkeley: University of California Press.

Strathern, Marilyn. 1990. *The Gender of the Gift: Problems with Women and Problems with Society in Melanesia*. Berkeley: University of California Press.

———. 2005. *Partial Connections*. Walnut Creek, CA: Altamira Press.

Stromberg, Joseph. 2012. "Why Did the Mayan Civilization Collapse? A New Study Points to Deforestation and Climate Change." http://www.smithsonianmag.com/science-nature/why-did-the-mayan-civilization-collapse-a-new-study-points-to-deforestation-and-climate-change-30863026/?no-ist.

Stucky, Mark. 2005. "He Is the One: The Matrix Trilogy's Postmodern Movie Messiah." *Journal of Religion & Film* 9 (2): Article 7. https://digitalcommons.unomaha.edu/jrf/vol9/iss2/7.

TallBear, Kim. 2016. "Beyond the Life/Not Life Binary: A Feminist-Indigenous Reading of Cryopreservation, Interspecies Thinking and the New Materialisms." In *Cryopolitics: Frozen Life in a Melting World*, edited by Joana Radin and Emma Kowal. Cambridge, MA: MIT Press.

Támez González, Silvia, and Rosa Valle Arcos. 2005. "Desigualdad Social y Reforma Neoliberal en Salud." *Revista Mexicana de Sociología* 67 (2): 321–356.

Taussig, Michael. 1987. *Shamanism, Colonialism, and the Wild Man: A Study in Terror and Healing*. Chicago: University of Chicago Press.

Terry, Edward, Ben Fallaw, Gilbert Joseph, and Edward H Moseley, eds. 2010. *Peripheral Visions: Politics, Society, and the Challenges of Modernity in Yucatan*. Tuscaloosa: University of Alabama Press.

Tharyan, Prathap, and Clive Adams. 2003. "Electroconvulsive Therapy for Schizophrenia." *Cochrane Database of Systematic Reviews*. Issue 2. Art. CD000076. http://cochranelibrary-wiley.com/doi/10.1002/14651858.CD000076.pub2/full.

Todd, Zoe. 2016. "An Indigenous Feminist's Take on the Ontological Turn: 'Ontology' Is Just Another Word for Colonialism." *Journal of Historical Sociology* 29 (1): 4–22.

Tozzer, Alfred M. 1941. *Landa's Relación de las Cosas de Yucatán*. Vol. 18 of *Papers of the Peabody Museum of Archaeology and Ethnology*. Cambridge, MA: Harvard University Press.

United Nations. 2006. Convention on the Rights of Persons with Disabilities. United Nations. https://www.un.org/development/desa/disabilities/convention-on-the-rights-of -persons-with-disabilities.html.

Varley, Emma. 2016. "Abandonments, Solidarities and Logics of Care: Hospitals as Sites of Sectarian Conflict in Gilgit-Baltistan." *Culture, Medicine and Psychiatry* 40:159–180.

Vasconcelos, José. (1979) 1997. *La Raza Cósmica/The Cosmic Race*. Baltimore: Johns Hopkins University Press.

Vergano, Dan. 2012. "Maya 'End of World' Is a Mistranslation." *USA Today*, December 13. https://www.usatoday.com/story/tech/2012/12/13/apocalypse-not-maya-end-of-world -a-mistranslation/1768143/.

Villaseñor Fajardo, Sergio, Alma Baena, Ricardo Virgen, Martha Aceves, Mayra Moreno, and Irma Gonzalez. 2003. "La Participación de la Familia del Paciente en la Hospitalización Psiquiátrica de 'Puertas Abiertas': Un Modelo de Atención Etnopsiquiátrica." *Revista de Neuro-Psiquiatría* 66:185–194.

Villegas, Omar. 2016. "There's a Crew in Mexico Rapping in Maya." *Mitú World*. https:// wearemitu.com/mitu-world/a-group-of-mexican-rappers-are-making-music-to-instill -pride-in-their-community/.

Viveiros de Castro, Eduardo. 2012. *Cosmological Perspectivism in Amazonia and Elsewhere: Four Lectures Given in the Department of Social Anthropology, Cambridge University, February– March 1998*. Vol. 1, Hau Masterclass Series, *Hau Journal of Ethnographic Theory*.

———. 2014. *Cannibal Metaphysics: For a Post-structural Anthropology*. Minneapolis, MN: Univocal Press.

Wachowskis, dir. 1999. *The Matrix*. Burbank, CA: Warner Brothers.

Warren, Kay B. 1998. *Indigenous Movements and Their Critics: Pan-Maya Activism in Guatemala*. Princeton, NJ: Princeton University Press.

Watanabe, John, and Edward Fischer, eds. 2004. *Pluralizing Ethnography: Comparison and Representation in Maya Cultures, Histories, and Identities*. Santa Fe, NM: School for Advanced Research.

Watters, Ethan. 2010. *Crazy Like Us: The Globalization of the American Psyche*. New York: Free Press.

World Health Organization (WHO). 1992. *The ICD-10 Classification of Mental and Behavioural Disorders: Clinical Descriptions and Diagnostic Guidelines*. Geneva: World Health Organization.

———. 2017. Global Health Observatory (GHO), country views.

INDEX

abandonment, 2, 26, 75; by family, 78, 121; reasons for, 81–82; zone of, 79–80, 81. *See also* social abandonment

abuse: patients as targets for, 71; within psychiatric institutions, 92–93; as reason for suicide, 74; vulnerability to, 55. *See also* sexual abuse

Agamben, Giorgio, 16, 80

agrarian reform program *(reforma agraria)*, 14–15, 34

aka pacha (indigenous temporality), 42, 176n. 7

Americanized Spencerism, 6

anachronism, 13

anti-psychiatry movement, 84, 86

Anzaldúa, Gloria, 40–41

Appadurai, Arjun, 96

bare life, 16, 80

Behold the Black Caiman (Bessire), 163

Bennett, Jane, 150

Bessire, Lucas, 163, 179n. 3

Bhabha, Homi, 16

Biehl, João, 80

biological psychiatry, 119

biomedicalization, 87, 114

biomedical models, 20, 91

biomedicine, 27, 69; confidence in, 135, 141; doctors embracing, 131

Bonfil Batalla, Guillermo, 67–68

borderlands, 40–41

Borderlands/La Frontera: The New Mestiza (Anzaldúa), 40–41

Butler, Judith, 48, 146, 152

Calderón Narváez, Guillermo, 7

capitalism, 13, 38

Cárdenas, Lázaro, 14–15, 34

Carr, E. Summerson, 69

Castañeda, La, 7, 13, 169

Caste War, 15

Castillo Cocom, Juan, 17, 34, 47, 164; ethnoexodus concept by, 42–44; performance role in writings by, 48

Catholic Church, 9

Chase, Arlen, 44–45

Christianity, 45

chronic patients *(crónicos)*, 69–70, 80

civic engagement, 9

class: clothing marking, 142; dimensions of race and, 23; as identity category, 176n. 4; importance of, in local identity, 35–36

Clemente Orozco, José, 11

clinical case-study session *(sesión clínica)*, 110–114, 178n. 2

clothing: as marking ethnicity, gender and class, 142; as protection, 145–146; transformative power of, 143–146

collective memory, 14, 34

colonialism, 7, 46, 177n. 11; current world order defined by, 169; establishments of, 103; neoliberalism, modernity and, 104; persistent strain of, 13. *See also* internal colonialism

coloniality, 16, 30–31; capillary functioning of, 82; as constitutive of modernity, 11–12; as defining characteristic of society, 103; definition of, 13; existence shaped by, 170; Grosfoguel arguments on, 40; identity, madness and, 42; as inescapable, 108–109; limits of notions of, 40; madness, modernity and, 56, 72, 87; Mignolo assertion on, 27, 40, 103

coloniality of power: change in dynamics of, 169; identifying, 108; manifestation of, 31; as mediator, 43

colonial matrix of power, 13, 26, 31, 71–72, 170; as constituted into being, 82; inner workings and reproduction of, 139; operationalization of, 114; power dynamics in, 44; psychiatric institutions as manifestation of, 156–157; social processes constituting, 82; Zona del Estar emerging from, 55

colonial violence, 16, 42

comorbidity designation, 69

CONEVAL, 39, 175n. 2

confinement: avoiding of prolonged, 155; deserving of, 7–8; madness and, 81; rights lost by, 42

continuity of care, 6, 95

conversion disorder, 144–146

corruption, 9, 169; culture of, 109; influence of, 68; as obstacle to modernization, 66–67; perpetuation of, 175n. 4

cosmic race, 34

crónicos (chronic patients), 69–70, 80

Culturas Híbridas (García Canclini), 12

culture: absence of, 10; of corruption, 109; lack of, 9; modernization and, 10; problem of, with patient compliance, 102; race blending with, 30; sense of loss from rejection of, 43

Cusicanqui, Silvia Rivera, 17

Davis, Elizabeth, 115–118

deception, 115, 116

decolonization, 16–17, 31

deinstitutionalization, 70, 79

Deloria, Vine, Jr., 148–151

delusions, 6, 125–127, 142, 155, 157–161

dementia, 7, 63, 128

Diaz, Porfirio, 6, 12, 169

Disability-Adjusted Life Year (DALY), 18

Disability Rights International (DRI), 2, 21, 75, 87, 92–93, 167

disease burden, measure of, 18

dispossession, subjugation, oppression and, 16

Dresden Codex, 50–53

Duncan, Whitney, 10, 98

economic reforms, 4, 97

education: Indigenous Education System, 99–100; intercultural model of, 45; reform for, 59

ejido system, 15

electroconvulsive therapy (ECT), 21–22, 84, 92–93, 126–127, 160–163, 166

emotion pedagogy, 98–99

Enlightenment, 86

entitlement, false sense of, 49

epistemic plurality, 41, 42, 80, 163, 176n. 9

esclavitud (slavery), 14–16, 34, 175n. 6

Esperanza, La (suicide prevention group), 60–61, 88, 107

ethics: of personal responsibility, 117–118; questions of, 24–25

ethnicity, clothing marking, 142

ethnoexodus, 42–44, 150, 177n. 10

ethnographic entrapment, 164; ethnographic refusal and, 47; Ixtab as iteration of, 54; Zona del Estar as entangled in, 46, 48

ethnographic gaze, 46

ethnographic refusal, 47

ethnopsychiatric model, 8

family: abandonment by, 78, 121; as allowed to stay with patients, 80; cohesion and strength of, 21; dysfunctional dynamics within, 111–113; failure of, 20; importance of unity of, 40, 63, 78; locating of, 75, 81; presence of, 18; psychiatric diagnosis made easier by, 129; role of, 8, 79; treatment options from support of, 130

Fanon, Frantz, 6, 16–17, 26; colonized psyche and, 27; The Wretched of the Earth by, 14, 55, 86; zones of being and nonbeing by, 41, 42

Ferguson, James, 7

Foucault, Michel, 10, 86, 109

Freud, Sigmund, 86

Fromm, Erich, 86–87

Frontera, La/Borderlands: The New Mestiza (Anzaldúa), 40–41

García Canclini, Nestor, 10–12

Garza, Mariana, 97

gender: clothing marking, 142; intersection of indigeneity and, 33–34

gender identity, 48

Gender of the Gift, The (Strathern), 141

Gledhill, John, 58

globalization, 96

Gone, Joseph, 17

Gonzalez, Irma, 61–62

González Casanova, Pedro, 41

Good, Byron, 18

governmentality, 96, 115

Grebenshikov, Boris, 3, 118

Grosfoguel, Ramón, 17, 26, 31, 40, 41

Güemez Pineda, Miguel, 20

Guerra de Reforma (War of Reform) (1858–1861), 11

Gupta, Akhil, 7

Hayden, Cori, 99, 119
health care workers: benefits for, 59; mobilization of, 58, 62
Health Insurance Portability and Accountability Act (HIPAA) (1996), 24–25
henequen monoculture, 14–15
heritage, 31, 34, 50, 177n. 13. *See also* Maya heritage
Hidalgo Model, 166–167
Hirose, Javier, 19, 150
homelessness, 71
Hospital Leandro León Ayala (Asilo Ayala), 6–7, 13, 84
huaches (Mexican foreigners in Yucatan), 9, 23
human rights: investigations into, 28, 38, 165; violations of, 2, 74, 92–93, 118, 179n. 3
hybridity, 11–12
hybridization, 12
hysteria, 7

identity: categories of, 23, 34, 36, 151, 176n. 4, 176n. 6; coloniality, madness and, 42; importance of class in local, 35–36; importance of verifying, 118–119; limits in categories of, 41; Maya culture linked to expression of, 55; *mestiza* as specific type of, 33; role of temporality in shifts of, 44. *See also* gender identity; indigenous identity; Maya identity
identity politics, 46, 50
iknal (physical presence in absence of physical body), 19, 150, 151
Import Substitution Industrialization (ISI), 12–13, 175n. 5
independence, 27
Independent Festival of Maya Culture, 45
indígena. See indigenous people
indigeneity, 11–12; fetishized notions of, 46; intersection of gender and, 33–34; madness, suicide and, 26; symbol of, 33; Zona del Estar, madness and, 42–43, 176n. 9
indigenismo, 34
indigenous identity, 33; complexities of, 40–42; decolonizing of, 31; flexibility of, and Zona del Estar, 56; mental health relationship with, 42; understanding of, 35. *See also* Maya identity
indigenous metaphysics, 148, 150

indigenous people: control over, 164; lack of respect for, 178n. 7; local understanding of, 31; modernity claim of, 41; portrayals of, 54; problematic relationship between society and, 103; worldviews of, integrated into psychiatry, 100
indigenous temporality *(aka pacha)*, 42, 176n. 7
indigenous thought, 151
inferiority (biological), 7
Informe Contra Idolorum Cultures (Sánchez de Aguilar), 50
institutionalization, 69–70, 166; doctors' interest in avoiding, 130; prevention of, 81; role of, in state policy, 71; trauma of, 91
Instituto de Seguridad Social de Trabajadores del Estado (ISSSTE), 63–65, 93
Instituto Mexicano del Seguro Social (IMSS), 3, 37, 63–65
insurance: cheating on schemes of, 26; continuity of care interrupted by, 95; market for private health, 93–94; moral dilemma of double enrollment for, 65–67, 177n. 3. *See also* Seguro Popular
integrative medicine, 97
interculturality *(interculturalidad)*, 27, 94; adoption of, 99; embracing principles of, 103; guidelines for, 100–102
internal colonialism, 41
International Festival of Maya Culture, 45
Inventing Ourselves (Rose), 10–11
invisible beings, 141–142, 163, 179n. 8
involuntary commitment, 20, 70; force necessary during, 90; isolation as factor in, 21; legal responsibility of institution as result of, 81; reasons for, 74
isolation, 21
Ixtab (suicide deity), 26, 50, 51–53, 54

Jenkins, Janis, 5, 10
Joseph, Gilbert, 9
Juarez, Benito, 11–12

Kahlo, Frida, 11

labor, 18, 59
Labyrinth of Solitude, The (Paz), 66
Landa's Relación de las Cosas de Yucatan (Tozzer), 50

Latour, Bruno, 141, 151, 179n. 2
lobotomy, 84, 126
locura. See madness
Lucero, Lisa, 44
Luhrmann, Tanya, 5, 113

madness, 4–8; boundaries pushed by, 170;
confinement and, 81; identity, coloniality
and, 42; indigeneity, Zona del Estar and,
42–43, 176n. 9; modernity, coloniality and,
56, 72, 87; as opportunity for shift in
temporality, 55; psychosis as heart of, 142;
space between sanity and, 13, 43, 71;
suicide, indigeneity and, 26; temporality
of, as understood through Zona del Estar,
71; as within zone of nonbeing, 42
Madness and Civilization (Foucault), 10
magical thinking, 10
magic modern, 141
marianismo, 54
Marín, Guillermo, 67–68
Marx, Karl, 86
materiality, 146, 148
Matrix, The, 82
"Maya," 26; as invented ethnic category, 47,
54–55; production of, 163–164
Maya culture, 29–30; efforts to revitalize, 48;
indigenous metaphysic within, 150;
interpretations of, 44–46; as linked to
expression of identity, 55; monetary value
of, 44; preservation of, 50
Maya heritage, 42, 46, 48, 53–56, 163–164
Maya identity, 46, 48, 163–164
Maya language, 16, 33; children losing, 56;
endangerment of, 46; training in, 22
Mayan Apocalypse, 26, 44–45
Maya people, 19; architecture of, 15; as
fetishized, 43; as mysterious, 45; as prone
to suicide, 34, 50–54
Mayer-Serra, Carlos, 8–9, 67
McCormick, Kenny, 29
medicalization, 6, 84
medical neglect, 37–38
medication, pharmaceutical: access to, as
difficult, 63–65, 128–129; doctors' reliance
on, 81; importance of dosing of, 77; as
necessary for schizophrenia, 73; overuse
of, 113; quality of life transformed through,
83–84; shortages of, 134

melancholy, 6
mental health care: availability of, 17–18, 93;
indigenous identity relationship with, 42;
obstacles to access, 95–96; public services
for, 3; symptoms linked to, 19; systems
available for, 19
mental illness: in children, 20–21; as
compatible with biomedical models of
care, 91; intelligence and, 111; local
interpretations of, 18–19; methods for
explaining individual cases of, 113–114;
physical illness distinguished from,
153–154; poverty relationship with, 39–40;
prevalence of, 17–18; processes of
assessment of, 105, 136–137; as stigmatized,
6; uniform representing, 144; violence
provoked by, 91–92; ways of understanding, 85–86
mestizaje, 12; frameworks of, 26; as modern
construct, 41; politics of, 32–33
mestizas, 41; as fetishized, 33–34; produce
sold by, 30
Mexican Renaissance, 11
Mexican Revolution (1910), 7, 72
Mexico Profundo (Bonfil Batalla), 67–68
Mignolo, Walter, 11, 16–17; borderlands
embrace of, 41; coloniality assertion of, 27,
40, 103
mobilization, of health care workers, 58, 62
modernism, 10
modernity, 4, 27, 40, 67; alternatives to, 17;
coloniality as constitutive of, 11–12; as
complex, 11; as destination, 8–9; equated
with whiteness, 6; indigenous people's
claim to, 41; madness, coloniality and, 56,
72, 87; neoliberalism, colonialism and, 104;
post-Enlightenment, 86
modernization, 6, 99; corruption as obstacle
to, 66–67; as deficient, 10–11
Morris, Stephen, 68

negotiation: diplomacy as basis for effective,
120; language importance in, 133;
relationships built through, 118; as strategy,
132; truth, orientation and, 116, 138–139
neoliberalism, 13, 58, 62, 87, 96, 99, 104
neoliberal subjectivity, 96, 116
nepotism, institutionalized, 58–59, 62
nerves (*nervios*), 19, 72, 94, 153–154, 176n. 8

neurosyphilis, 7
New Age religions, 45
North American Free Trade Agreement
    (NAFTA), 12–13, 99
Nuijten, Monique, 58

objects: as having spirits, 149–150; as
    repositories of relationships, 141;
    transformative force of, 147
One Flew Over the Cuckoo's Nest, 2, 4
ontological colonization, 163
ontologies, 148–151, 179n. 8
oppression, subjugation, dispossession
    and, 16
orientation: lack of, resulting in zone of
    nonbeing placement, 130; levels of, 129;
    questions utilized to determine, 137–138;
    truth, negotiation and, 116, 138–139

Pan-Maya movement, 34–35
Partido de Acción Nacional (PAN), 13, 49, 60
Partido Revolucionario Institucional (PRI),
    13, 59–61
party politics, 59–61, 82, 168
pathology of normality, 87
patients, mental health: as abuse targets, 71;
    admittance process for, 92; bill of rights for,
    116–117; collaboration between doctors
    and, 115–116; as committed after arrest, 90;
    consent from, 25–26; continuity of care for,
    95; culture as problem for compliance of,
    102; developmentalist discourse observed
    in, 124; experiences of, 73–78; family as
    allowed to stay with, 80; as manipulative,
    106; privacy for, 24–25; progress of, 170;
    psychiatric institutions used as escape by,
    106–107; refuge sought by, 85; ruptured
    relationships characterizing illness
    experiences of, 153; as stripped of
    self-determination, 80; subjugated
    knowledges held by, 96–97; support
    network importance for, 75; tactics used
    by, 69; trust lacking in, 119; uniform
    opinions of, 143–144. *See also* chronic
    patients
Paz, Octavio, 4, 11, 66
Peña Nieto, Enrique, 9, 66–67
performance, 48
pharmaceutical revolution, 83–85

Popol Vuh (Maya creation story), 47
positionality, 23
positivism, 12
poverty, 4; defining levels of, 175n. 2; as
    identity category, 36, 40; mental illness
    relationship with, 39–40; powerlessness
    from, 38; social belonging and, 35–36; as
    source of pain, 39
privatization: of oil, 59; of resources, 12
privilege, white, American, 23
protectionism, 12–13
protests, by hospital staff, 57–58
psicoeducación, 98–99
psychiatric diagnosis, 97; delusions analyzed
    for, 158–160; developing skills for, 178n. 2;
    family as helpful in, 129; psychoanalytic
    approach to, 131; socialization leading to,
    116; truth as critical for, 115
psychiatric emergencies, 91
psychiatric institutionalization, 4
psychiatric institutions, 2; abuse within,
    92–93; failure of, 38; federal takeover and
    remodel of, 165–168; human rights
    violations plaguing, 118; internal processes
    of, 88–89; as manifestation of colonial
    matrix of power, 156–157; monastery
    similarities with, 107–108; navigating all
    spaces of, 132; patients' use of, as escape,
    106–107; physical conditions of, 89, 93,
    178n. 7; as resembling general hospitals, 85;
    social processes within constraints of, 72;
    as subject to local politics, 108
psychiatric power, in colonial matrix of
    power, 115
psychiatry: biomedicalization of, 87;
    diagnosis not primary goal of, 113; doctors'
    depth of interest in, 130–131; history of, 6,
    87, 180n. 2; as mechanism of social
    regulation, 86; reputation of profession of,
    84; as situated social practice, 56;
    worldviews of indigenous people
    integrated into, 100
psychopharmacology, 87
psychosis, 23, 108; confusion surround-
    ing, 122; experience of, 92; as heart of
    madness, 142; patients' experience of, 25;
    subjective experience of, 139; triggers for,
    154–156
psy sciences, 10, 86

Quijano, Aníbal, 13–14, 41, 71, 82

race: as biological, 32–33; culture blending
    with, 30; dimensions of class and, 23.
    See also cosmic race
racialization, 41
racism, 13, 35, 103
Ramos, Jorge, 8–9
rationality, 10, 116, 138, 152, 170
reforma agraria (agrarian reform program),
    14–15, 34
rehabilitation, 10, 81, 87, 166–167
relationality, 152–154
remittances program, 99
responsibility, 27; for being healthy, 99; ethics
    of personal, 117–118; fostering of personal,
    98; as foundation of neoliberal person-
    hood, 119
Reyes Heroles, Federico, 8–9
Ríos, Gabriela, 41
Ríos Luviano, Saúl, 47–48
Ríos Molina, Andrés, 6–8
Rivera, Diego, 11
Rivera Cusicanqui, Silvia, 30, 35, 40–41, 47,
    176n. 7
Rose, Nikolas, 10–11, 86, 96

Salinas de Gortari, Carlos, 3–4, 97, 99
Sánchez de Aguilar, Pedro, 50
sanity: fragility of, 6; space between madness
    and, 13, 43, 71; as within zone of being, 42
Saturno, William, 44
schizophrenia, 18, 39, 73, 76, 91, 104–105, 120
secularism, 11
Seguro Popular, 3, 38, 57, 63–66, 93, 97
self, composition of, 19
self-actualization, 27, 116
self-determination, loss of right to, 42, 80
self-injury, 68–69
self-sufficiency, 27, 84, 97–98
sesión clínica (clinical case-study session),
    110–114, 178n. 2
sexual abuse, 55, 79
Simpson, Audra, 17, 46
Siqueiros, David Alfaro, 11
slavery (*esclavitud*), 14–16, 34, 175n. 6
Smith, Daniel, 67
social abandonment, 8, 70–72, 80
social belonging, poverty and, 35–36

social death, 80
social environment, symptoms aggravated by,
    108, 127
social integration, 84–85
socialist humanism, 86
social processes, 26, 71; as constituting
    colonial matrix of power, 82; within
    constraints of medical institutions, 72
social regulation, psychiatry as mechanism
    of, 86
sociology of absence, 42, 176n. 9
de Sousa Santos, Boaventura, 14, 26, 41, 42
Spanish language, 23–24, 42–43
spirits, recognition of, 20, 148
spirituality, 107–108, 147–148
Strathern, Marilyn, 141
strikes, 28, 167–168
subjectivities: as conflicting, in health care
    system, 99; expressions of, 11; materiality
    intersection with, 146; as neoliberal, 27. *See
    also* neoliberal subjectivity
subjugation, dispossession, oppression and, 16
suicide, 34–35, 88; abuse as reason for, 74;
    aftermath of attempted, 107–108; attempt
    to commit, 39, 91, 179n. 5; as cultural rather
    than structural problem, 55; experiences of
    spirituality and, 147–148; madness,
    indigeneity and, 26; Maya people as prone
    to, 50–54; rates of, 49–50; as relational, 154.
    See also Esperanza, La; Vida es Bella, La
suicide deity (*Ixtab*), 26, 50–54
symptomology, 7, 112
symptoms: descriptions of, 111; emulating of,
    106; hiding of, 155–156; linked to mental
    health, 19; recognition of, 20–21; social
    environment aggravating, 108; transforma-
    tion of, 157

TallBear, Kim, 148–151
Taussig, Michael, 130, 141
temporality: madness as opportunity for shift
    in, 55; of madness as understood through
    Zona del Estar, 71; of psychiatric wards, 43;
    role of, in identity shifts, 44; Zona del
    Estar characterized by, 151, 156. *See also*
    indigenous temporality
Tlatelolco massacre, 14
Todd, Zoe, 151
tourism, 26, 30, 44–45

Tozzer, Alfred, 50
traditional medical practices, 19, 94, 96
treatments: family support creating options
    for, 130; process of developing, 112–113; use
    of combination of types of, 94
truth, 27, 80; as critical for psychiatric
    diagnosis, 115; as enshrined in violence,
    139; medical intervention ability to
    obliterate false, 127; negotiation, orienta-
    tion and, 116, 138–139

uniforms, 2, 103, 143–144, 150
United Nations Convention on the Rights of
    People with Disabilities (CRPD), 75

Vasconcelos, José, 4
Vida es Bella, La (suicide prevention
    organization), 59–60
Villaseñor Fajardo, Sergio, 79, 100
violence, 3, 12; mental illness provoking,
    91–92; as structural, of capitalism, 38; as
    symbolic, 163–164; truth as enshrined in,
    139. See also colonial violence

Vita (Biehl), 80
Viveiros de Castro, Eduardo, 148, 151, 163

War of Reform (Guerra de Reforma)
    (1858–1861), 11
wildlife, as omen, 20
withdrawal, dangerous results of, 98
Wretched of the Earth, The (Fanon), 14, 55, 86

Yucatan Comisión de Derechos Humanos del
    Estado de Yucatan (CODHEY), 74

Zapatista movement, 14, 17, 99
Zona del Estar, 177n. 10; characterization of,
    42; as conceptual tool, 26; as emerging from
    colonial matrix of power, 55; as entangled in
    ethnographic entrapment, 46, 48; flexibility
    of indigenous identity and, 56; indigeneity,
    madness and, 42–43, 176n. 9; temporality
    characterizing, 151, 156; temporality of
    madness understood through, 71
zone of being, 41, 42–43, 55
zone of nonbeing, 41–43, 55, 80, 130

ABOUT THE AUTHOR

BEATRIZ M. REYES-FOSTER, PHD, is associate professor of anthropology at the University of Central Florida. A sociocultural and medical anthropologist, she has published numerous articles on mental health, suicide, and Maya identity and culture in Mexico.